SHUNGITE

SHUNGITE

Protection, Healing, and Detoxification

REGINA MARTINO

Translated by Jack Cain

Healing Arts Press
Rochester, Vermont • Toronto, Canada

Healing Arts Press
One Park Street
Rochester, Vermont 05767
www.HealingArtsPress.com

Healing Arts Press is a division of Inner Traditions International

Originally published in French under the title *La shungite: énergie de vie* by Éditions Ambre,
    Geneva, Switzerland
First U.S. edition published in 2014 by Healing Arts Press

*Note to the reader: This book is intended as an informational guide. The remedies, approaches,
and techniques described herein are meant to supplement, and not to be a substitute for,
professional medical care or treatment. They should not be used to treat a serious ailment without
prior consultation with a qualified health care professional.*

Library of Congress Cataloging-in-Publication Data
Martino, Regina, 1960– author.
  [Shungite. English]
  Shungite : protection, healing, and detoxification / Regina Martino ; translated by Jack
Cain. — First U.S. edition.
      pages cm
  Includes bibliographical references and index.
  ISBN 978-1-62055-260-5 (pbk.) — ISBN 978-1-62055-261-2 (e-book)
  1. Minerals—Therapeutic use. 2. Minerals in the body. 3. Detoxification (Health) I.
Title.
  RM258.5.S3413 2014
  613.2'85—dc23

                                                                        2013032992

Printed and bound in the United States by Versa Press

10   9   8   7

Text design and layout by Virginia Scott Bowman
This book was typeset in Garamond Premier Pro with Trajan Pro used as the display
    typeface
Photographs by M.- D. Vrac

CONTENTS

ACKNOWLEDGMENTS

I wish to thank my husband, Christophe, for his support and invaluable assistance, Stéphane Cardinaux for his collaboration and thoughtful advice, and Christel Barbier and David Buffault for their participation in the initial bioenergetic lithotherapy research.

And I pay homage to Mother Earth for her rich, astonishing, and inspiring mineral resources.

MY FIRST ENCOUNTER WITH SHUNGITE

My first encounter with shungite goes back to 2006 when I was collaborating with Stéphane Cardinaux during his training sessions in Paris. Stéphane is a practitioner and trainer in geobiology and bioenergy. He has a degree in architecture from the École Polytechnique Fédérale de Lausanne and is the founder of the school Génie du Lieu (meaning "genius of place," as in the Latin *genius loci*) in Lausanne, Switzerland. We took advantage of these times in order to refine the results of the work each of us had been doing in bioenergy and geobiology. One of the subjects of our investigation involved the ultimately harmful effects of electromagnetic waves, the measurement of these effects, and the quantification of their energetic impact on living things.

One evening, after a day of training, we met Alexander Rusanov, a Russian geologist who was seeking Stéphane's assessment of a system Rusanov had brought from the Ukraine. Rusanov placed some little round plastic boxes in our hands, then asked us to be aware of what we felt and to tell him about our first impressions. I'll never forget the stunned look I exchanged with Stéphane. The effect was really something!

The first sensation we felt was that of a lightning-fast impact that spread up through the body, followed by a great expansion of life energy along with a beautiful feeling of substantiality or energetic density! We immediately had the intuitive sense of having touched something important, something monumental with respect to our ongoing research. Of course, we immediately asked this geologist what it was all about. What was inside those innocent-looking little boxes that had such an immediate and strong effect?

They contained *shungite*—a word we had never heard before and which meant nothing to us. What on earth was shungite?

Our curiosity was intense and we absolutely had to know more. Above all we wanted to run a series of tests on this substance to find out if our first impressions would stand the test of bioenergetic measurement. Stéphane and I began testing these boxes containing shungite—which, by the way, were called Spinor—he in Switzerland and I in Paris, each with a team of researchers. The results of several months of research were surprising for us because not only did shungite offer protection against the negative effects of electromagnetic waves (the reason our geologist friend was interested) but it also had other very positive effects for the energetic system as a whole.

During this time I was in the midst of conducting a more detailed study of the bioenergetic effect of crystals with two other bioenergetic researchers, Christel Barbier and David Buffault, and I wanted to find some natural shungite to include in the tests that were in progress.

In 2006 and 2007, there was no mention of shungite in any

published works on lithotherapy and none of the stores selling stones and crystals in France carried it. I finally found a few fragments for sale on the Internet in the United States and I waited impatiently for my parcel to arrive. I still remember the moment I held that tiny, 0.5 cm (less than a quarter of an inch) piece of natural shungite in my hand for the first time; a real nugget of energy!

From that moment on I haunted the mineral shows looking for this exceptional substance and I questioned all the Russian salespeople that I met. Making contact wasn't easy. Certain salespeople in the business knew about shungite, but they hadn't yet realized there was a market for this strange, silvery-black mineral.

After numerous tests, we verified that our initial intuition was right. We had found something *natural to protect life.*

We still had to find enough quality shungite in order to recommend it and sell it to clients who consulted us on questions of geobiological expertise or bioenergetic assessments. Prevailing upon a young Russian man whose grandfather was a geologist, I finally managed to convince him to go and look for good quality shungite directly in a mine in Karelia, a region in the northwest of Russia bordering Finland and the White Sea. (See the color insert, plate 1, for a photo of a shungite mine.)

It was not until 2008 that I was able to make quantities of this powerful mineral available for the benefit of my clients. In the meantime, I increased the number of tests, adding more and more detailed procedures using the different qualities and forms of shungite that were capable of affecting individuals—as well as locales and even plants. The more our research progressed, the more encouraging the results were. In fact, they generated a lot of enthusiasm and I realized that a mineral that concentrated all these properties without any dangers could be commercialized and marketed, beyond just training seminars, to all my clients in geobiology and bioenergetics.

In the fall of 2009 shungite was, as yet, little known in France even though our research work and the work of other researchers began to expand and become known. This was when I set up my own sales site: www.shungite.fr. Since 2009, shungite's popularity has continually increased and now you can find it easily in France and the United States. (See the resources section at the end of this book.) Many users have already experienced it and are very happy with it.

I invite you on a voyage in which we will discover shungite through a number of disciplines—a bit like being in high school—including geography, history, geology, and biology. Each discipline will provide us with key information so we can better understand shungite's beneficial qualities; even though many practical applications remain to be discovered. Of course, you can jump ahead right away to the more "energetic" or practical chapters; however, reading about the more scientific aspects will more completely answer your questions about the unique properties of this extraordinary stone.

1

WHAT IS SHUNGITE?

In order to start on the right foot, I must add a couple of lines on the pronunciation of the word *shungite*.

The name is derived from the name of the Karelian village of Shun'ga, where the mineral was first discovered. *Shungite* is pronounced to rhyme with *kite*.

THE DIFFERENT TYPES OF SHUNGITE

It's important to keep in mind that shungite in its natural state contains varying amounts of organic carbon. For this reason you will find stones being marketed under the name *shungite* that have different appearances. The explanation is very simple: they contain differing quantities of carbon. Following are the three qualities of shungite that are usually found.

Type I Shungite (Silver Shungite)
Type I occurs as a black, vitreous mineral with a semimetallic, silvery shine. It contains 98 percent organic carbon. This is the most scarce form since it accounts for only 1 percent of all

shungite that is found. It occurs in very narrow veins having a maximum width of 40 cm (16 inches). It can be easily identified because of its conchoidal fractures. Ocre-colored inclusions are jarosite, a basic sulfate of iron formed from the oxidation of pyrite (see color insert, plates 2–4, for photos of type 1 shungite). Sometimes, in marketing it, this type of shungite is called *crystalized* because of its naturally faceted appearance but this term is incorrect since shungite is an amorphous mineral and never crystalizes into any shape.

Composition

Carbon = 98%

Nitrogen, Oxygen = 0.9%

Hydrogen = 0.3%

Ash content up to 0.8%

Type II Shungite (Black Shungite)

Type II occurs as a black mineral. This is the kind of shungite most often used to make objects because, unlike type I, it can be easily shaped and polished (giving it a brilliant shine). (See plate 5 in color insert.) It contains 50 percent to 70 percent organic carbon.

Composition

Carbon = 64%

Nitrogen, Oxygen = 3.5%

Hydrogen = 6.7%

Ash content up to 3.3%

Type III Shungite (Gray Shungite)

This occurs as a gray-colored mineral and contains 30 percent to 50 percent organic carbon.

Composition

Carbon = 30%

Silicon dioxide = 56%

Water = 4.2%

Aluminum oxide = 4%

Iron oxide = 2.5%

Potassium peroxide = 1.5%

Magnesium oxide = 1.2%

Sulfur = 1.2%

Calcium oxide = 0.3%

Sodium oxide = 0.2%

Titanium dioxide = 0.2%

There are stones containing a lower percentage of organic carbon. These are termed *shungite rock* instead of *shungite*.

DEFINING SHUNGITE

If we were to provide a mineralogical definition for the purest type of shungite (type I), we could say that shungite is a 98 percent carbon, noncrystalline, nongraphite, structurally heterogeneous, vitreous, black mineral with a semimetallic shine.

The mineral is identified as *shungite* in Walter Schumann's *Gemstones of the World* (a definitive reference work in the field of gemology).

2

SHUNGITE IN HISTORY

Even though the marketing of shungite in Western Europe is gaining momentum, we shouldn't hail it as a magic and auspicious discovery capable of saving all beings on the planet. It seems more accurate to me to turn directly to the history of Russia, acknowledging that Western countries are not necessarily acquainted with the uses of shungite that have been known and recognized in Karelia for centuries. The fact that fullerenes* were discovered and named based on experiments in space laboratories should not be taken as some kind of reappropriation by the West. The Karelians have used fullerenes for centuries without knowing what they were.

After all, for countless generations our ancestors have used the healing properties of herbs, springs, and stones without having any scientific concept of pharmacology, biochemistry, or atomic and molecular structure. Many intuitive discoveries of the past,

---

*A fullerene is a molecule formed entirely of carbon in the form of a hollow sphere, ellipsoid, or tube. They will be discussed in more depth in chapter 4, "Shungite and Fullerenes."

even the remote past, have made possible enormous progress in present-day scientific medicine.

This mineral, formed billions of years ago, has been known for thousands of years by local people in the region of Lake Onega (the Russian part of Karelia). Archeological research has uncovered numerous very ancient human settlements in this area.

As people followed the retreat of the glaciers in the last ice age (around 9,000 BCE), nomadic tribes of hunter-gatherers gradually settled in Karelia. These people left behind petroglyphs and rock paintings dating back four thousand to nine thousand years and containing images that very often remain mysterious. The rock carvings at Lake Onega, dating from

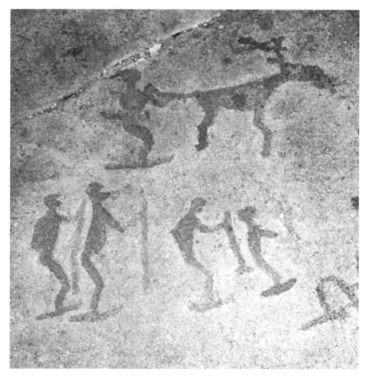

Petroglyphs of Karelia

the Neolithic era, notably portray mythological scenes directly related to nature, the seasons, and the elements. Certain themes evoke aquatic birds (their interpretation remains uncertain), mythological creator gods, the progression of seasonal change, migratory patterns, and the transmigration of souls. The Heavenly Elk, the Elk Man, and the Great Mother are also to be found among these petroglyphs. The carvings are found mainly on the eastern shore of the lake which has the richest sites of Finno-Ugrian rock carving.

Several archeological digs around the lake have brought to light dwellings and sacred sites (labyrinths, sacred stones, burial sites) dating to about 6,000 BCE. Lake Onega is sacred to the Sami shamans. It's a place of power where the very pure waters are a silent witness to their private ceremonies.

Much later, beginning in the fourteenth century, numerous orthodox churches and convents were built in this area, notably the famous Kizhi Pogost, the parish precinct on the island of Kizhi (fourteenth century) that contains the Church of the Transfiguration (1714), which was built without a single nail or any metallic element. This church has been designated a UNESCO World Heritage site.

Similar to what took place in Western Europe, these Russian churches were not erected in this location haphazardly. In addition to the fact that they lie on trade routes and on sites of great beauty, they draw benefit from the sacred sites that the ancients had chosen for their energetic properties.

Russian chronicles of the seventeenth and eighteenth centuries bear witness that shungite had already been in use for healing at that time. The first official written mention of the healing powers of shungite takes us back to the reign of Ivan the

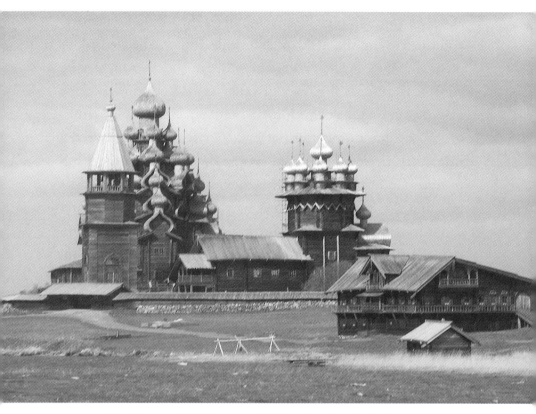

*The famous Kizhi Pogost on Kizhi island on Lake Onega
in the Republic of Karelia, Russia*

Terrible and his son Feodor I, which saw the end of the Rurikid dynasty. Shungite was not known then by its current name. This black rock was considered to be a local "slate" and was particularly famous for the very pure spring water that sprang forth from it.

Boris Godunov (regent and brother-in-law of Feodor I) had himself elected tsar in 1598 and, in order to avoid having his legitimacy to the throne challenged (because he was only an elected tsar), he tried to distance himself from the Romanov family's influence. He sent the only remaining Rurikid still alive, Feodor Nikitich Romanov, his wife Xenia Romanova, and their young son Mikhail into exile, forcing them to adopt monastic vows. Feodor Romanov was sent to Poland where he adopted the monastic name of Filaret. Xenia Romanova became a nun, assuming the name Martha, and sequestered in a hermitage at Tolvuya, to the north of Lake Onega, where she hovered near death, depleted by privations and the cold. Upon the death of Boris Godunov (in 1605), his oppressive regime loosened its grip and the local peasants, taking pity on her, saved her and cared for her with water from a spring that had miraculous properties (the shungite spring). Once she recovered her health, Martha/Xenia was reunited with her son Mikhail from whom she had been separated for many years. This took place before he returned to Moscow to put an end to eight years of political turmoil and to have himself elected tsar in 1613, taking the place of the usurpers who had preceded him.

Mikhail (Michael I) became the first tsar of the Romanov dynasty, which was to reign for three hundred years until the revolution of February 1917. This anecdote about shungite has come down to us because the death of Xenia/Martha would have brought about significant changes in Russia's history. To commemorate the recovery of this noble lady, the spring was named the Spring of the Princess. The spring was quickly forgotten in Moscow, however, and the miraculous water returned to anonymity as a source of help and healing, benefiting only the inhabitants of the neighboring villages.

Not until the reign of Peter the Great of Russia does shungite reappear in the annals of history.

In 1714, in a factory established by the tsar for the production of copper near Lake Onega, legend has it that workers who

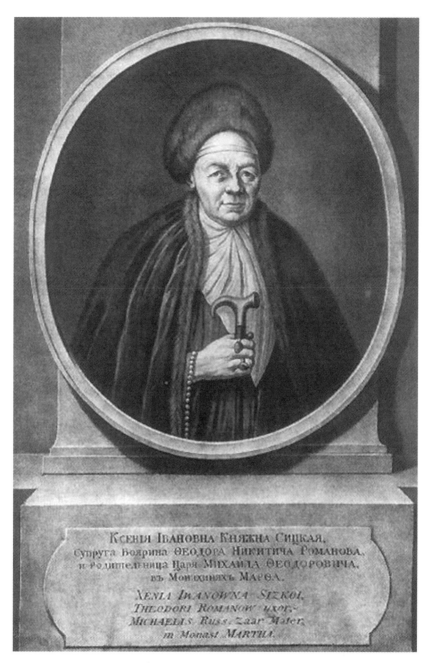

Xenia Romanova as the nun Martha

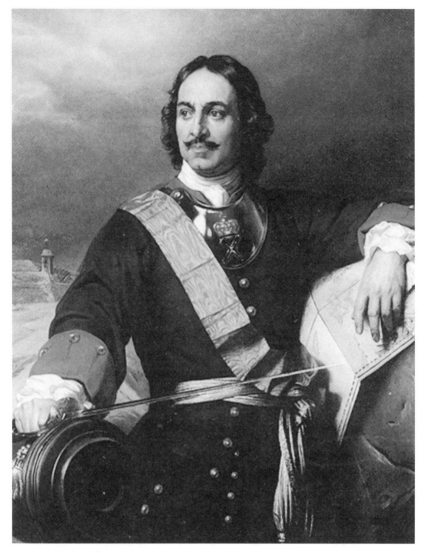

Peter the Great of Russia

were poisoned or fell seriously ill because of the ore they were processing could be healed in three days with the "living water" from a nearby spring. Peter I ordered an investigation of the spring, which flowed out from a shungite deposit. These investigations clearly showed the extraordinary properties of this water in healing illnesses such as scurvy and liver problems, among others.

After having spent some time at a Belgian thermal spa on the advice of Dr. Robert Areskin, his advisor and friend, the tsar ordered the construction of the first Russian spa at Konchezero on the shores of a small lake near Lake Onega. The spa he created was called Martial Waters. Three wooden palaces (destroyed in 1780 by fire) were built for the tsar, his family, and his court as well as homes and inns for the patients and for the staff. The tsar also had the Church of Apostle Peter erected between 1720 and 1721.

An article written during this period, entitled "Inquiry on the True Properties of the Martial Waters of Konchezero," contained nine brief descriptions of the illnesses treated by the waters from this spring. In the 1720s, Peter I returned with his family many times for treatment using the martial waters. Having experienced the unique antiseptic properties of water that had been in contact with this black stone and knowing that it conferred great vitality to those who drank it, Peter the Great ordered by decree that each one of his soldiers was to carry a piece of shungite (the name was to appear later—at this time it was still called slate rock) in their packs and to put it in their water flasks so as to always have pure, disinfected water, thus avoiding the dysentery that so often plagued armies of those times.

After the death of Peter the Great, the thermal spa closed down and was forgotten by all except the local people. It was only in the 1930s that new medical studies of the water were carried out. They demonstrated that the level of ferrous oxide (79.7 mg/l) was greater than that of similar waters of worldwide renown from the spas of Marienbad or Carlsbrunn. However, the Second World War halted all plans to once again build a spa.

The 1960s saw a resurgence of interest in shungite with the construction of a new spa and new clinical research, but once again these studies remained confined to the local level. This research however has garnered a greater exposure since the discovery of fullerenes in shungite. Chapter 5, entitled "Shungite Properties and Effects on Health: Twenty Years of Russian Research," will describe the results of more recent research; scientifically demonstrating the beneficial qualities of shungite.

3

THE ORIGIN AND GEOGRAPHY OF SHUNGITE

Getting to shungite's origins takes us very far back in time.

Our solar system was formed about 4.6 billion years ago. Earth was formed in this far away time by the accretion* of gas and dust and from the shock of planetesimals (small planets) emerging from the protoplanetary nebula. The Earth was originally a ball of congealing lava, resulting from multiple bombardments by large blocks of matter and forming as a result of internal movement such as complex contractions, the rearranging of component materials, and volcanic activity. Then the Earth cooled and by about 300 million years after its formation (4.3 billion years ago) its surface was covered by protocontinents and oceans. This was primitive Earth.

Between 3.8 and 3.5 billion years ago the formation of the

---

*Accretion designates the capture by a star of matter under gravitational influence.

Earth's crust and creation of the first mountain ranges took place. During this era we see the appearance of the first signs of life at a molecular level in the ocean.

The first elements to carry life were proteins (amino acids); the simplest molecules imaginable. After proteins, bacteria formed that were composed entirely of membranes and devoid of nuclei. They are called prokaryote cells—unicellular beings that already have the essential attribute of life: a strand of DNA.

These first building blocks of life were cyanobacteria (also called blue-green algae) and stromatolites. The first stromatolites, which were found at the North Pole and at Pilbara (in western Australia), are the first irrefutable trace of the existence of bacterial life. They date to 3.5 billion years ago.

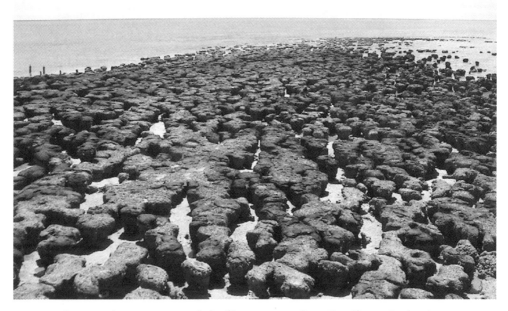

Stromatolites or stromatoliths ("stone carpets" in Greek)—rocky limestone structures that build into cauliflower-like mountainous formations. They are composed of microorganisms, such as cyanobacteria, that precipitate bicarbonate into calcium carbonate.

Geological time has been subdivided chronologically in order to better delineate and understand the history of the Earth. The Precambrian era in the geological calendar is the longest since it extends from the formation of the Earth 4.6 billion years ago up to 550 million years ago (89% of the Earth's geological time). This era includes the eons named Archean, Hadean, and Proterozoic. We are presently in the following eon (the fourth eon) called Phanerozoic, the eon that has witnessed an explosion of macroscopic life.

In looking at the scale represented in the diagram below, we can see the enormous duration of the Precambrian era compared to the subsequent geological eras. The whole history of human-kind is included in the last line on the right: a simple, minuscule little line at the right margin of the whole diagram.

Shungite was formed from organisms living at the beginning of the Proterozoic eon (2–2.2 billion years ago). The remains of unicellular prokaryote organisms of this period built up and mixed with mud and silt to form layers of sediment. According to Russian geologists, these sediments accumulated over a vast area of the Karelian craton (created during the Archean eon), which is made up of a volcanic continental rift, in an environment of

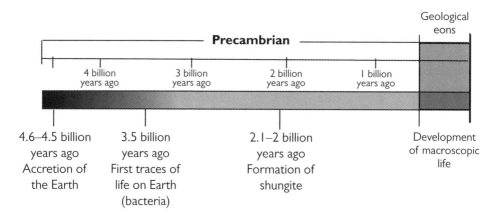

lagoons rich in brackish water (and therefore saturated with minerals and salts).

The combination of volcanic activity with an environment of lagoons fostered the development of organic life. The decomposition of these bountiful microorganisms led to the formation of a significant sedimentary layer—kerogen. The sediments sank slowly into the soil and little by little were transformed into rock through the effect of compression (tectonic plate movement). With the rise in temperature (due to subterranean volcanic activity and geothermal heat), the organic materials were then transformed into simpler substances—hydrocarbons in the form of petroleum or bituminous shale, as well as coal.

There is a very significant difference between shungite and petroleum or coal. The timescale is completely different. Petroleum and coal were formed between 300 and 600 million years ago, that is about 1.5 billion years later than shungite.

The kerogen of the Karelian craton would then have had the time and the right environmental conditions to turn from a liquid or fluid state into a solid state through a slow process of petrification. This process was also responsible for the creation of the natural molecular structure of the fullerenes, as the carbon atoms combined spatially into the form of a soccer ball. The vast area over which shungite is spread in Karelia is a result of its dispersion and migration due to geological movement (tectonic plate movement).

Other hypotheses have been developed. Some scientists think that the fullerenes present in shungite resulted from lightning strikes in storms. This theory is strongly disputed though because of the high level of fullerenes found in the Karelian deposits of shungite. It has been proven that lightning can in fact create fullerenes (see chapter 4 on fullerenes), but only in trace quantities.

Other scientists have promulgated the hypothesis of a meteoric origin for the fullerenes. It is true that, at 2.4 billion years old, the oldest recorded meteorite crater on Earth is the Suavjärvi crater found about 50 km (31 miles) from Lake Onega. And, as we will see later in the chapter on fullerenes, fullerenes have been detected by astronomers in a nebula. We cannot then rule out the possibility that a meteorite could have been among the environmental factors that contributed to the creation of fullerenes in shungite. However, no scientific study is currently able to prove it.

Shungite is only found in one place on Earth—in the Russian part of Karelia. The deposit of shungite extends over a vast area of nine thousand square km (3,475 square miles), situated northeast of St. Petersburg, quite near Lake Onega. Lake Onega, at about half the size of Lake Ontario, is the second largest lake on the European continent, after Lake Ladoga, Russia. It has a surface area of 9,616 square km (3,713 square miles) and includes more than 1,600 islands or islets. This lake-dotted region is a basin of tectonic origin, hollowed out by glaciers and presenting a magnificent countryside of lakes, rivers, streams, and forests.

Shungite can be found on the surface following erosion and convection. However, it is generally found in the depths of the Earth, sometimes several hundred meters below the surface. The main accumulations of shungite are concentrated for the most part in nine layers, ranging in thickness from 5 meters (16 feet) to 120 meters (400 feet). The thickest layer is number six (counting up from the lowest).

One of the first studies to specifically name shungite was set up between 1880 and 1886 by Alexander Inostranzeff (1843–1919), a Russian geologist and paleontologist. As mentioned earlier, the name *shungite* was taken from the name of a village near one of the first extraction sites: Shun'ga.

4

SHUNGITE AND FULLERENES

Until recently it was thought that carbon occurred in only two allotropic forms—allotropy being the ability of a substance composed of only one type of atom (a simple substance) to exist in different molecular or crystalline forms—amorphous carbon and crystalized carbon. The second of these two includes three known natural forms: diamond, graphite, and lonsdaleite—the last of these having been discovered in 1967. These substances differ in their atomic structure.

For example, in the case of diamond, each carbon atom is located at the center of a tetrahedron with the four closest atoms at its apexes. This particular atomic structure is what makes diamond the hardest substance known.

In the case of graphite the carbon atoms form a hexagonal ring. As the rings multiply they create a solid and stable lattice resembling a beehive. These sheets are placed one over the other in layers that are weakly linked together. This structure defines the specific properties of graphite: it doesn't hold together and separates easily into little flakes. The 2010 Nobel Prize in Physics was awarded to the first researchers who were able to "peel down" graphite to a layer only one atom thick. This very solid atomic lattice is called graphene.

The existence of giant molecules of carbon was a hypothesis that was a by-product of the calculations of quantum physics. In 1970 Eiji Osawa, a Japanese researcher at the Toyohashi University of Technology, hypothesized that a complete form of carbon in the shape of a soccer ball could theoretically exist. In the 1980s a series of laboratory experiments were conducted to detect the existence of stable structures containing sixty carbon atoms. On September 4, 1985, Harold Kroto, James R. Heath, Sean O'Brian, Robert Curl, and Richard Smalley discovered C60. Shortly afterward they observed the first fullerenes; leading to the award of the Nobel Prize in Chemistry to Kroto, Curl, and Smalley in 1996.

The name *fullerene* originates from a different source. It was derived from the surname of Richard Buckminster Fuller (1895–1983), an American engineer, architect, inventor, and writer. He is known for having discovered and named the structural principle of tensegrity, or tensional integrity, which is the ability of a structure to stabilize through the interplay of the forces of tension and compression based on the distribution and balancing of the mechanical constraints throughout the structure. He is also known for his works on synergetics, for his participation in the Gaia hypothesis, and especially for being the creator of the architectural concept of the geodesic dome, which he applied in the construction of the United States pavilion at the Montreal Exposition in 1967 (Expo 67).

The geodesic dome that Fuller conceived is an exact replica of the structure of fullerene C60.

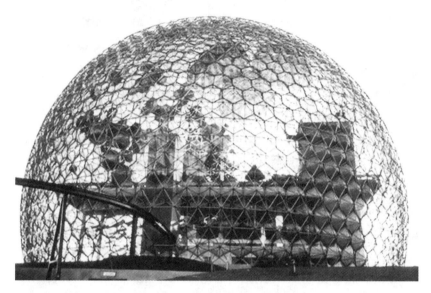

Buckminster Fuller's geodesic dome

Fullerenes then are a new form of carbon discovered in the laboratory. The smallest stable fullerene (its pentagonal rings are not beside each other) bringing together sixty carbon atoms (C60) is composed of twenty hexagons and twelve pentagons in the shape of a soccer ball. There are other fullerenes such as C70, C72, C76, and C84.

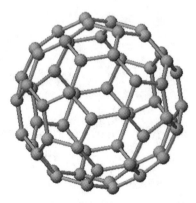

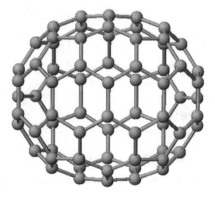

C60 fullerene   C70 fullerene

Since their discovery, chemists have tried to produce larger quantities of fullerenes in order to be able to more easily study their unique properties. It was only in 1991 that techniques for obtaining fullerenes were fully developed and obtaining a gram of fullerenes is still difficult. In 1991, the journal *Science* called the fullerene the "molecule of the year" and declared that it constituted "the discovery most likely to shape the course of scientific research in the years ahead."

Fullerenes have unusual behavior in certain physicochemical reactions, probably because of their symmetry and because they constitute an envelope that may ultimately contain other molecules or ions in their centers. Unlike diamond or graphite that cover their external surface with hydrogen atoms, fullerene molecules are not constrained to do that. For example, it has been established that a natural fullerene will allow certain free radicals to react with it, attracting them to its surface without losing its symmetrical balloon shape (C60). We will see in a later chapter that this characteristic has already led to medical applications. Certain researchers conclude that the pentagonal structure of C60 fullerenes shows that fullerenes are organic molecules, or even a molecular crystal that constitutes a link between organic and inorganic substances.

FULLERENES IN NATURE

Chemists have conducted studies to determine if it would be possible to discover fullerenes in nature. A Russian geochemist discovered the first proof that the molecules of carbon called fullerenes occur naturally on the Earth. Using a high resolution electron microscope to examine shungite, Semeon J. Tsipursky noticed that certain images contained the same range of black and white circles that characterized the micrographic centers in samples of synthetic fullerenes.

Tsipursky, in collaboration with Peter Buseck, geochemist at Arizona State University at Tempe, found fullerenes and C60 and C70 in shungite. Buseck then sent a variety of samples to Robert L. Hettich, a chemist at Oak Ridge National Laboratory in Tennessee. Using a mass spectrometer, Hettich analyzed them without knowing that they came from a natural source. He confirmed the presence of fullerenes. Researchers reported this discovery in the journal *Science* in July 1992.

In 1998, other researchers in India confirmed the presence of fullerenes in shungite: G. Parthasarathy, R. Srinivasan, M. Vairamani (National Geophysical Research Institute, Hyderabad), and K. Ravikumar and A. C. Kunwar (Indian Institute of Chemical Technology, Hyderabad).

In 2006 a study was conducted by N. I. Alekseev, D. V. Afanas'ev, B. O. Bodyagin, A. K. Sirotkin, N. A. Charykov, and O. V. Arapov and reported in the *Russian Journal of Applied Chemistry* on the formation mechanism of fullerenes in shungite. Their results were as follows:

The formation of particles of fullerenes in shungite involves a certain number of morphological characteristics that are distinct from particles resulting from chemical products and arc syntheses.

1. The particles have an empty cavity that may be filled with water or traces of water.
2. There are no metallic nanoclusters encapsulated inside the layers of fullerenoids.

3. The layers of fullerenoids around the nanoparticles can have topological intervals; that is, the surface generally does not have a fullerene character in the strict sense of the word.

4. Particles of fullerene exist both in type III shungite containing 40% of aluminosilicates and type I shungite in which the concentration of aluminosilicates is no higher than a few one hundredths.

Other chemists have carried out studies showing that fullerenes can be found in nature. They have discovered for example that they are present in soot and in certain combustion conditions, in fulgurites (glassy rocks formed when lightening hits the ground), and also in interstellar space. The discovery of C60 and C70 fullerenes in a cloud of cosmic dust in a planetary nebula was made by Jan Cami in 2010 using NASA's Spitzer telescope.

Fullerenes have also been found in meteoric impact craters (notably the Sudbury crater in Canada and the Allende and Murchison meteorites in Hawaii). Scientific studies are under way at present to determine if the fullerenes come from the meteorites themselves or if they were created by its impact. This information has led scientists to speculate on the role that fullerenes may have played in the creation of life on Earth. Gases may in fact be easily trapped inside these hollow molecules. A research group (Luann Becker, Jeffrey L. Bada, Robert J. Poreda, and T. E. Bunch) has already found traces of a form of helium in fullerenes extracted from the Sudbury crater. It is theoretically possible that, if the fullerenes have a stellar origin, they could have contributed both the carbon that is indispensible to life and the volatile substances that led to producing the conditions necessary for planetary life.

Peter R. Buseck declared in 2010, "There is abundant evidence that the mineralogical world is wondrously complex and full of surprises. We prefer to retain an open mind about the extent of fullerene occurrences in the geological environment [rather] than to make possibly premature conclusions based on the limited data at hand."

ARTIFICIAL FULLERENES

Since their discovery, fullerenes have been subjected to a certain number of molecular manipulations in the laboratory consisting of modifications to their form. Researchers have been able to create nanotubes of fullerenes that are useful for a wide range of applications in the field of nanotechnology. There has also been experimentation with the addition of certain atoms and molecules. The stable molecular structure of a fullerene combined with interspersed atoms has given birth to a whole family of superconducting compounds.

On this topic we need to mention an experiment conducted on the influence of fullerene molecules on cellular membranes. A computer simulation, using many computers networked together, was able to demonstrate that, at least in this virtual world, the molecules of fullerenes do not puncture the cellular membranes in a mechanical way. Instead they dissolve through it and then reassemble inside the cells. This research took place in the field of nanotechnology and only refers to fullerenes in the form of nanotubes. It has not been carried out using a simulation of natural fullerenes.

In the scientific press recently there have been warnings about the toxicity of fullerenes. However, it is important to note that this is based on research conducted with fullerenes that have been created in the laboratory. This scientific research manipulates the molecular structure of the fullerenes, as we have mentioned before, in order to find applications in nanotechnology and super-conductivity. The research is not about natural fullerenes such as those found in shungite.

The conditions of the artificial creation of fullerenes, including C_{60}, are such that they do not take into account spin direction in the formation of the molecules. Also, these artificial molecules do not contain the same gases and atoms in their hollow interior (at the center of the soccer ball) that natural fullerenes do.

I had an opportunity to test a small quantity of these synthetic fullerenes and I can confirm their toxicity from the bioenergetic point of view. I subjected a small quantity of artificial fullerenes—less than a gram of C_{60} and C_{70}—to bioenergetic tests with several individuals. The results indicate a loss of 55 percent of the person's vital energy field and a decrease of 65 percent in the emanation of the first chakra, whereas I remember that the same tests using the natural fullerenes contained in shungite showed an increase of 100 percent in the person's vital field.

5

SHUNGITE PROPERTIES AND EFFECTS ON HEALTH

Twenty Years of Russian Research

Shungite is not a passing fancy. It's true that it has come upon us with the force and speed of a lightning bolt, but the history of its relation with humankind has endured for hundreds of years or even more as indicated by numerous sacred Neolithic sites in the area of Lake Onega.

Russian scientists have been studying it for a long time, but the Second World War interrupted this research for many years. Since the 1960s however, doctors and Russian researchers have established new research protocols in order to test the validity of the properties of shungite on human health. It is worth mentioning that the isolation of the Soviet world from Western influence meant that for decades it was spared the overpowering domination of multinational pharmaceutical companies. Thus, Russian researchers were able to profit from their relative isolation by developing scientific research independently while retaining the disinterested curiosity of legitimate scientists. In Europe and the

United States it is more difficult to find serious and independent medical studies aimed at proving the viability of natural remedies that cannot be turned into a profitable monopoly.

The first scientist to prove that the specific properties of shungite were due to the presence of fullerenes was Grigory Andrievsky working at the Institute of Therapy at the Ukrainian Academy of Medical Sciences. His studies were followed by those conducted by a team directed by Nina Kolesnikova. These studies and the results of numerous other research studies led by various scientists were presented at a conference dedicated to shungite in October 2006 in Petrozavodsk.

GRIGORY ANDRIEVSKY'S RESEARCH

This scientist sought to identify the active principle that had created such widespread passionate interest in the martial waters and other products containing shungite that were currently being used by spas and in home remedies in Russia's northwest.

Using various procedures, Professor Andrievsky precipitated out the various aqueous solutions available to create a base, called an *Andrievsky solution,* containing a significant concentration of fullerenes. Andrievsky noticed, however, that the fullerenes that had been isolated and concentrated in this way did not constitute a remedy or medication in the accepted meaning of those terms. It was therefore impossible to assign the shungite fullerenes to a pharmacological classification. His conclusions indicate that natural fullerenes act on a systemic level and not as a treatment for an illness. They act as an adaptogen operating both at the cellular level and at the level of the whole human body.

It is important therefore to understand that shungite (and

particularly the natural fullerenes that it contains) is not a medication. In order to better understand one of the beneficial actions of natural fullerenes, we first need to review the nature and purpose of antioxidants.

Antioxidants are substances that for the most part inhibit the process of oxidation and peroxidation of free radicals. Under ordinary life circumstances, free radicals are relatively scarce and their pathological effects on the cells of the body are to a large extent offset by the ingestion of antioxidants found in a balanced diet. These antioxidants are found in vitamin C, vitamin E, beta-carotene, and certain enzymes contained in tannins, among other things.

A deficiency of antioxidants or an excess of free radicals can result in the destruction of cells and lead to heart attacks, neurodegenerative diseases, and cancer. When the body is subjected to particularly harmful factors, such as radiation, we see a multiplication of free radicals leading to a weakening of the body's systems and requiring the provision of more antioxidants to rebalance the whole. A deficiency in antioxidants is also part of the aging process.

Professor Andrievsky's team concluded that aqueous solutions of natural fullerenes are among the most powerful antioxidants known today. Natural fullerenes not only have the ability to reduce the concentration of free radicals as no other antioxidant can but their action is stronger and it lasts longer. And, as the researchers explain, this is true because the mechanism by which natural fullerenes act is different from other antioxidants. The molecule of a classical antioxidant combines with a free radical to form a resultant harmless molecule through a mechanism of neutralization. In contrast, natural fullerenes act as catalyzers.

Thanks to its soccer-ball shape, a molecule of natural fullerene attracts free radicals that end up stuck to it, covering its entire surface. Having numerous free radicals side by side on a fullerene base leads to their molecular transformation into a neutral compound. At the same time, a fullerene does not lose its molecular composition and continues to attract free radicals.

According to the work of Andrievsky, fullerene molecules are a permanent catalyzer in the recombining of free radicals, even in very reduced dosages and over a period of several months. The conclusions of this work extend even further and identify the following complementary effects:

- Natural fullerenes derived from shungite normalize cellular metabolism, increase enzymatic activity, stimulate the ability of tissues to regenerate, increase the resistance of the body's cells, possess anti-inflammatory properties, and foster the exchange of neurotransmitters.
- Natural fullerenes also act against toxins and can neutralize toxins present in the body. Specifically, active fullerenes in the liver reduce toxicity levels and foster the elimination of certain toxins present in this organ.
- In the same way, certain internal toxins resulting from burns and from some other necrotic processes are eliminated, which speeds up the healing of this type of wound.

This research has also shown that fullerenes have an effect on excessive exposure to heat. When the body temperature reaches certain thresholds of heat (high fevers for example), proteins present in the body undergo destructive molecular modifications. The presence of natural fullerenes in the body significantly increases the stability of biomolecules that have been exposed to an excess of heat. The Russian scientists quickly found a practical application of this in the field of oncology.

The Ukrainian Academy of Medical Sciences conducted experimental protocols on volunteer cancer patients who had undergone sessions of radiation therapy. Detailed blood analyses were conducted on these patients before, during, and after their treatment with radiation therapy; both for the group that had received shungite water and for a control group. The doctors found that blood levels returned to normal in two weeks following the radiation in patients who had taken shungite water, whereas it took an average of three to four months for the values of those in the control group to return to normal levels.

THE WORK OF NINA KOLESNIKOVA AND HER TEAM

Dr. Nina Kolesnikova is in charge at a sanatorium near Moscow that specializes in cardiology, but also treats diabetes, hypertension, and infectious diseases. She decided to use shungite in the treatment of the following illnesses:

- High blood pressure
- Joint pain issues
- Osteoarthritis
- Chronic nasal infections and respiratory tract infections
- Diabetes mellitus and diabetic angiopathy
- Pathology of the gastrointestinal system
- Psoriasis

Patients exhibiting hypertension, psoriasis, and joint problems were given a shungite bath for ten to fifteen minutes every day. The doctors observed a stabilization in the condition of these patients, an increase in their well-being, and a desire to return to a physically active life.

For patients with joint issues and psoriasis, a heated shungite paste between 1 and 2 centimeters thick was applied to the affected area over several successive days for twenty to thirty minutes each time. The doctors observed a reduction in lesions, a lessening of pain, an increase in joint mobility, and a decrease in joint stiffness.

The report on the work of this medical team also contains the following information which we quote here:

> Shungite was also used as a mouthwash for sore throats, stomatitis, and periodontitis and gave good results.
>
> Shungite water (carbonate, sulfate, chlorine, magnesium, sodium) was used with diabetic patients. The treatment improved their well-being, stabilized the metabolizing rate of carbohydrates, and reduced the level of skin irritation and lesions.
>
> Treatment with shungite water was also seen to be significant for digestive system illnesses. Shungite water was administered in 100 ml dosages on an empty stomach and was used for chronic colitis, gastritis, pancreatitis, and cholecystitis. The shungite water had a toning and anti-inflammatory effect. It reduced bloating, acid reflux, and returned stools to normal.
>
> Shungite was also used directly in the form of a natural stone to massage the feet. This foot massage doesn't have

any direct contraindication, but does require the individual's choice as to the length of the procedure. Measuring the blood pressure before and after the procedure was a precondition for this massage. The absence of any significant change in direction of the rising or falling arterial pressure meant that the procedure was well chosen. The procedure lasted an average of two to five minutes. The impact on the reflexology areas on the foot contributed to an improvement in the blood supply to organs and tissues. Such a procedure had a positive effect on degenerative joint disease, on lumbosacral radicular (radiating) pain, and on osteochondrosis.

In concluding this report, the medical team would like to report that it is in favor of continuing the use of shungite given its positive effects on the patients, but also because it made possible a reduction in the amount of medication needed by these patients.

A SCIENTIFIC CONGRESS TITLED "SHUNGITE AND THE PROTECTION OF HUMAN LIFE"

This congress was held in October of 2006 in the town of Petrozavodsk in Karelia, and was the first congress of its kind entirely devoted to shungite.

Many researchers participated in it; each one presenting their evidence and results of their research. At this time the following effects of shungite have been identified:

- Antibacterial (Krutous, 2002; Rysev; Khadartsev, 2002)
- Antiviral (Khadartsev, 2002)

- Immunostimulant, in the absence of a response to the stimulation of the Ig E (Immunoglobulin E) (Khadartsev, 2002)
- Anticancer agent (Khadartsev, 2002)
- Anti-inflammatory/antioxidant (blocking the peroxidation of lipids) (Krutous, 2002; Rysev)
- Antihistamine (Rysev and others)
- Protection from ionizing and noniodizing radiation (Kurotchencko, Subbotina, and others, 2003)

Here are a few extracts:

Experimental Medical Use of Shungite at the White Springs Sanatorium at Petrozavodsk

The White Springs sanatorium of Petrozavodsk has been operating for twenty years as a spa with facilities capable of accommodating 150 persons. The techniques used in this spa are mainly hydrotherapy with mineral baths, fangotherapy (mud baths), ozone therapy, and shungite therapy.

Since 2001, the spa has been offering several treatment methods that involve shungite:

- Concentrated shungite water for external use (mouthwash, inhalation, body wrap)
- Shungite paste for local application
- Mixture of shungite in the mineral baths

More than 1,500 individuals have taken shungite treatment at the spa.

Application of shungite paste is used in treating osteochondrosis, radiculitis, and arthritis—445 individuals have been treated with an average of nearly ten interventions per stay.

Shungite baths are used for circulatory system illnesses—615 individuals have been treated with an average of eight baths per person.

Treatments with concentrated shungite water are used for chronic illnesses: respiratory and ENT (ear, nose, and throat) illnesses. These procedures have been given to 481 individuals, with an average of ten sessions per treatment. In the course of shungite treatments no secondary effects have ever been observed.

In the observation and follow-up of these procedures, the following positive effects have been observed:

+ Increase in the range of motion of the joints, reduction of swelling, and lessening of pain associated with illnesses of the musculoskeletal system (with four to eight applications of shungite paste)
+ Elimination of allergic skin reactions (hives) with two to three baths or the application of lotions of concentrated shungite
+ Elimination of occurrences of acute rhinitis after two or three inhalation procedures of concentrated shungite
+ Normalization of arterial pressure after six or seven shungite baths for patients with vascular disease
+ Reduction in juvenile acne in young patients with the use of concentrated shungite

In addition to medical usage, the spa also employs shungite to enhance general well-being by filtering swimming pool water and by additional purification of tap water using shungite filters. This considerably improves the quality of the water used in cooking and aids in the preparation of medicinal plants.

Based on the preceding information, we can draw the following conclusions regarding the use of shungite for medical purposes:

+ The use of mineral products based on shungite is effective in the prevention and treatment of disease.

+ Shungite can be used in spa treatments.

+ Mineral preparations based on shungite are not subject to restrictions based on the age of the recipient and can be used in regular baths and in mud baths.

+ The domestic and industrial use of shungite for filtration greatly improves the quality of tap water, which supports the use of shungite in the preparation of plant-based decoctions, teas, and in washing produce.

+ Production of filters containing shungite for use in the treatment of water for swimming pools will improve the color composition as well as the physical and microbial quality of the water.

The Use of Shungite Paste for External Application in Patients Suffering from Osteoarthritis

Osteoarthritis mainly affects women aged forty to sixty, but in recent years there has been both a significant increase in incidence of the disease, with sometimes serious symptoms, seen in persons aged thirty-five to forty-five and in the incidence of osteoarthritis in men (Going, 1991; Okorokov, 1997; Chirkin, 1993). This is a disease involving the degeneration and destruction of cartilage in the joints with a subsequent proliferation of bony tissue leading to joint deformation.

The development of medical nanotechnology, including the use of shungite in the treatment of osteoarthritis, opens up new possibilities in resolving difficulties in the treatment and prevention of this disease.

The aim of this study is to determine the usefulness of shungite paste used externally with patients exhibiting osteoarthritis in various areas of the body. The study was conducted in the sanatorium, known as *Beautiful,* located in the Belgorod area of Russia.

The conclusion of this study was that the use of shungite paste for osteoarthritis is a reliable and effective treatment that is characterized by a quicker and more in-depth improvement than from medication and physiotherapy combined. This suggests that shungite paste is an effective treatment for osteoarthritis and we recommend that it be introduced in treatment and rehabilitation programs for patients exhibiting this pathology.

Application of Shungite-Based Treatments for Illnesses That Involve Respiratory Tract Obstruction

Infectious diseases of the lower respiratory passages and bronchial asthma are challenging for internal medicine. The development of nanotechnology, including the use of shungite in the treatment and healing of asthma opens up new possibilities.

This study was conducted at the Beautiful sanatorium, in the Belgorod region. It involved the observation of 154 individuals ranging in age from eighteen to eighty who were suffering from bronchopulmonary disease.

A preparation based on a solution of shungite at a concentration of 0.10 mg/ml was given to patients suffering from various bronchial obstruction conditions. The solution was administered by inhalation for a period of ten minutes, with a volume of 5 ml of solution inhaled. After seven to fourteen inhalation sessions per day it was observed that the shungite has a bronchial dilation action of a quality at least equal to the classical bronchial dilation medications. Shungite can also be used in the following clinical situations:

- Prevention and treatment of the bronchial obstruction syndrome in patients suffering from chronic obstructive pulmonary disease (COPD)
- Prevention and treatment of asthma
- Reevaluation of the treatment of patients in these categories in order to get the conditions under control quickly and to reduce the amount of medication

Analysis of the literature and clinical experience suggests that shungite has an important role in the treatment of respiratory disease and in the treatment of bronchial obstructive disease. However, everything is not completely clear. Complementary studies are essential to helping develop new approaches for treatment, rehabilitation, and prevention of these diseases.

Evaluation of the Treatment of Hospitalized Patients Suffering from Cardiovascular Disease Using a Room Coated with Magnesium-Shungite

The following is an excerpt from a study done by A. I. Kalinin, M. J. Semkovich, and A. V. Yakovlev:

At the present time, the positive properties of shungite are continually reaffirmed and its usage continues to expand.

Shungite compounds have been used successfully in medicine in the treatment of diseases of the musculoskeletal system, diseases of the upper respiratory passages, and of the digestive tract. There are many reports concerning unguents, creams, and pastes based on shungite that have anti-inflammatory properties and are effective in the treatment of dermatological conditions. Positive results from the use of medications made from shungite in combination with other therapeutic factors have been demonstrated.

A new application of shungite involves using it as a construction material in the decoration and fitting out of health care establishments.

A mixture of magnesium and shungite (components of a construction plaster for which a patent has been sought following encouraging health and epidemiological assessments) was used in the construction of a special room in the clinic of the Voennomeditsinskoy Academy, a health care hospital.

In order to neutralize geological irregularities such as fault-zone anomalies, this room was coated with a shungite mixture to make it a self-contained, microecological zone devoid of magnetic properties due to its shielding against electromagnetic radiation and its "correction" of any geomagnetic anomalies.

Studying the effectiveness of treating cardiac patients in a hospital room fitted out with magnesium-shungite was quite interesting. The study's case-control protocols were followed with eighty-four patients suffering from coronary heart disease and hypertension (the average age was 62.5). Fifty-four patients constituted the main group and thirty others were in the control group that received standard treatment. The diagnostics were confirmed by clinical data, laboratory tests, and functional methods. The control parameters were measured daily until the patient's discharge from the hospital (after 14 to 19 days). Upon admission and at discharge, each patient's quality of life was evaluated using a questionnaire that included subjective data (cardiac pain) and objective data (laboratory data and blood pressure), as well as other variables such as their length of hospital stay.

The results of these studies were significant with regard to the length of hospital stay.

+ In the study group of patients suffering from congenital heart disease, the stay was 14.3 days (compared with 18.4 in the control group).
+ For patients suffering from hypertension the two results were 15.5 and 19 days, respectively.

The average difference was from 3.5 to 4 days. The lab work (biochemical blood analyses) did not show a significant difference between the two groups.

The results of the psychophysiological research tends in the direction of favoring the use of magnesium-shungite rooms. In general, the effect of the magnesium-shungite construction materials on the patient's central nervous system was positive. Thus, the simple sensorimotor response time in those questioned was significantly shorter in the magnesium-shungite group ($P<0.05$). The results obtained show an improvement in the level of functioning of these patients' central nervous system.

The ratings on all tests of quality of life also showed

significant improvement compared to the control group—emotional expressivity, pain, energy, sleep, and more.

In summary, the room clad with the magnesium-shungite compound represents an undeniable advantage in achieving therapeutic improvement with cardiac patients. It can be incorporated in general cardiac practice as well as in cardiac intensive care units in medical establishments. An additional factor in obtaining general clinical results may be improvements in the potentiation of the interaction with medications.

Kalinin, Semkovich, and Yakovlev's research findings continue:

In 2006, we added a collection of elements to the sungite room that were designed to increase our patients' relaxation: comfortable armchairs, sofas, relaxing music, fountains, paintings, soft lighting, and cushions as well as some additional shungite accessories designed to reinforce their medical treatment.

We measured the electromagnetic field levels in the room and controlled those levels before and after equipping the room with shungite. And we received authorization to make use of the room.

Starting in May 2006, we included in our treatment program the opportunity to spend time in this shungite room.

In order to study patients who were affected by their visits to the shungite room, we conducted an analysis with an IES-01 computer. The survey was conducted twice for each patient—before and after visits to the room, for each of ten sessions. The study was conducted using an electroacupuncture scanner designed to evaluate the screening and treatment of the various systems of the body.

We examined a group of twenty patients.

Group Structure

By age:

- 20% of the patients were under sixty
- 80% were over sixty

By sex:

- 20% men
- 80% women

By condition:

- 30% hypertension
- 30% osteochondrosis
- 20% coronary heart disease
- 10% asthma
- 10% rheumatoid arthritis

Conclusions on the Effects of the Shungite Room

After analyzing the results of the survey, we concluded that after ten sessions the energy level of the human body had changed with the effect that internal self-regulating mechanisms were activated:

- 40% of the patients showed a harmonization of energy
- 40% of the patients showed a weak rebalancing process
- 20% of the patients showed regression

In studying the relationship among the energy channels, we found that in 50% of the patients there was a breakdown in communication among the channels:

+ 80% of the breaks in connections among the channels of energy studied either disappeared or were considerably diminished after ten sessions in the shungite room
+ 20% of the connections among channels studied were new

The program that analyzes the results of the measurements taken includes a diagnostic section based on the work of the internal organs of the organism's overall system:

+ 60% of the cases showed a significant decrease in the number of conditions diagnosed
+ 20% of the cases showed no change in this number
+ 20% of the cases showed new conditions diagnosed

During the whole course of the study, we monitored the blood condition parameters before and after the procedure, which revealed a stabilization of arterial pressure during their stay in the shungite room. Significant changes in cardiac rhythm were also recorded.

Having begun to use the shungite room, thanks to a small group of patients, we have obtained initial positive results and we have established a program designed to continue our testing of the use of this treatment room by using the IES-01 computer to ensure follow-up of the treatment results.

A SHUNGITE ROOM IN BESLAN

The town of Beslan in North Ossetia (in the Russian Federation) sadly became infamous following the taking of hostages and the massacre of hundreds of people in September 2004. The terrorists had targeted a school and the children who survived were traumatized by images of indescribable suffering and by the violent deaths of many of their friends and companions. The psychological trauma inflicted on the children and also on the parents was at a horrific level.

In 2006 a shungite room was constructed in Beslan, near the new school. The children and parents were invited to use this shungite room to help improve their psychological health.

Psychiatrists noted that after a few sessions, children who were extremely introverted and disturbed began once again to make drawings with bright colors, sunshine, and flowers. And several children learned to smile once again.

Of course, sessions in the shungite room were only one element among a number of measures taken by psychiatrists and psychologists in the course of their handling of this situation.

There are several other shungite rooms. Among the oldest is one at Petrozavodsk in the White Springs sanatorium and there is another at the Military Academy of Medicine in St. Petersburg. The latter, constructed in 1996, has been used with a lot of success by numerous patients who experienced excellent results in terms of a reduction in the duration of medical conditions, some of which were very serious such as diabetes and various respiratory tract pathologies.

6

BIOENERGETIC
RESEARCH ON SHUNGITE

Since 2006 we have been conducting experiments on shungite in all of its forms using bioenergetic tests. The results have been so promising that even now we continue to formulate new protocols to further develop the research and to respond to user questions in the following domains: electromagnetic protection, natural therapies, geobiology, and agriculture.

In chapter 7, "Practical Applications," I will provide advice that comes directly from my experimentation.

BIOENERGY
AND BIOENERGETICS

Every living being constantly interacts with its environment by emitting electromagnetic and etheric emanations. It is the etheric emanation that corresponds to life energy, or bioenergy.

Bioenergy forms around the physical body in a series of successive layers that are characterized by increasing energetic density or concentration and that are contained one within the other like Russian dolls.

Bioenergetics is the subtle science that studies these fields. It also studies the emanation of the subtle centers called the *chakras* and other subtle parameters manifested by the energetic body of living beings. Tradition teaches us that every living being has a vital field emanating from the energetic body. The energetic body is made up of a distribution network of vital energy, or life energy, that includes the chakras and the meridians as well as an envelope that protects the physical body.

We will only be examining phenomena external to the physical body—the vital field and the chakras. These energetic fields move out infinitely like the circular waves that form on the surface of the water when you throw a pebble in a pond. The stationary waves form what is called the *vital field* and this field is used as a reference point in bioenergetics. It extends outward from the physical body to a distance of between five and eight feet (in 80% of the people who are measured).

The vital field is made up of a series of sublayers which always follow the form of the physical body and define its energetic concentration. Besides these parallel layers, there is a perpendicular partitioning, a series of planes, three of which are especially relevant as parameters for measurement: the vertical plane, the horizontal plane, and the lateral plane.

The vital field will almost immediately increase or decrease the moment there is a change in the person's immediate environment. The closer the change is to the person, the more the effect will be felt in the energetic body. When the disturbance is permanent, the vital field remains reduced and this can lead to the appearance of a physiological problem.

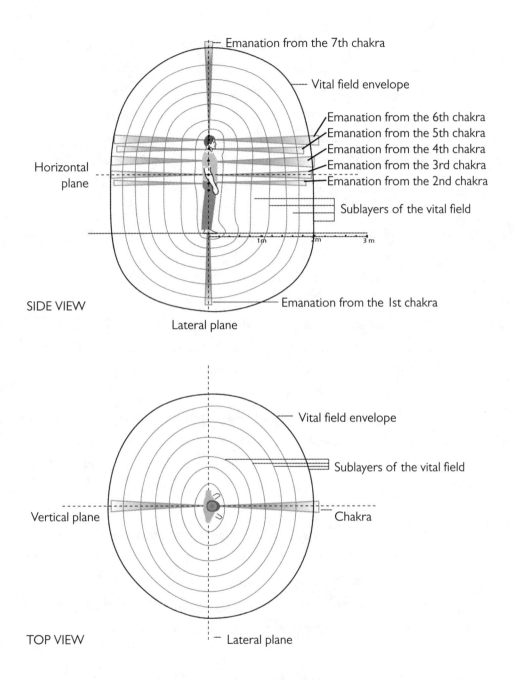

The vital field and the chakras.

The size of the vital field can vary considerably from one person to the next. It depends largely on the healthiness of the lifestyle, the general state of physical health, the level of consciousness, and environmental influences. Experience shows that absolutely everything has an effect on the vital field—our food, the water we drink, the various materials that make up the places we frequent, forms and colors, electromagnetic radiation, the geology of the Earth, the air we breathe, our thoughts, our emotions, the materials and colors of our clothing, the people around us, and more.

One other parameter that needs to be taken into account in order to understand the energetic system is the emanation of the chakras. The chakras are the main doorways of the subtle body. Their name comes from Sanskrit and means "wheels" or "discs." Although the transmission of this knowledge comes to us mainly from ancient India, the subtle centers have been known in various forms since ancient times. They have always been part of the teaching of spiritual masters and were used by the warriors of various traditions. The chakras can be defined and understood in various ways:

- Communication gateways for energetic exchange with the world (moving in and moving out)
- Our multidimensional connection (at different frequencies)
- The principal points of interconnection among the physical, emotional, mental, and spiritual bodies

In particular, Indian tradition describes seven chakras that are called *main chakras*. Recently, with the spread of yoga and Indian esoteric knowledge, this system of seven chakras has been adopted in numerous energetic disciplines and is widely used in lithotherapy.

The information that we collect in measuring the emanation from someone's chakras tells us about the quality of their relation to the world and about the seven planes or domains that each chakra governs energetically.

Movement of the Horizontal, Vertical, and Lateral Planes

The horizontal plane is the midpoint separation between the upper and lower portions of the vital field envelope. This plane passes through the navel and tells us about the cosmic and telluric balance in the person. It shifts when the field receives information coming from high vibrations or from low vibrations. And it moves back into place once this information has been integrated by the energetic body.

The lateral plane is not much used in bioenergetic tests of material because it indicates the person's subtle relation to time. The plane is positioned along the profile of the body (aligned with the ears) and represents the present. The part in front of the plane represents the future and the part behind it represents the past.

The vertical plane, like the horizontal plane, is very useful in testing the influence of materials and radiations on the energetic body. This plane divides the envelope of the vital field in two parts: the left and right halves of the body.

Movement of the vertical plane indicates disturbances in the energetic system due to an external influence (or an internal influence in the case of thoughts and emotions). This plane moves only to the left, which is explained by the levorotary (left rotation) molecular structure of all living or natural things. What influences this plane, and in doing so disturbs the overall vital field, are left torsion fields (see text box) produced by anything synthetic and artificial. This would include nonnatural electromagnetic radiation, the pulsed waves of cell phones, radiation from microwave ovens, and also, less forcefully, materials such as plastics and synthetic molecules. Most medicines, as well as many food supplements, are made up of synthetic molecules.

Torsion Fields

Élie Cartan (1869–1951), a French mathematician, carried out work on the interaction of algebra, geometry, and the analysis of complex bodies. Today his research is considered to be very advanced although it was slow to be recognized and remains relatively unknown. Notably, he provided mathematical tools for Riemannian geometry and for the theory of relativity. He developed a classification of symmetrical spaces and discovered the spinor, a vector that allows rotation of space to be expressed bidimensionally. His work, which later moved into the field of quantum physics, was taken up by Russian researchers, especially Nikolai Aleksandrovich Kozyrev (1908–1983). Kozyrev developed a theory about the existence of a spiral field or torsion field created by the form of an object or by the spin of elementary particles as defined in quantum physics (characterizing the behavior of the field associated with a particle under the effect of the symmetry of rotation of space). For example, torsion fields underlie the out-moving spirals of a seashell and the shape of a DNA molecule. A torsion field can have a right rotation (as in DNA) or a left rotation. Research conducted by the Russian scientist Vlail Kaznacheyev at the Institute for Clinical and Experimental Medicine at Novosibirsk has demonstrated that right rotation fosters life, whereas a torsion field that has left rotation has a negative effect on cells. Pulsed-wave radiation such as Wi-Fi and DECT (Digital Enhanced Cordless Telecommunications) generate left torsion fields.

The reality of the existence of torsion fields is still being debated. It is an innovative field of scientific research that is just beginning to be explored and needs further investigation.

Movement of the Planes of the Vital Field and Homeostatic Balance

All the planes of the vital field move based on incoming information. At the same time, the energetic system as well as the physical body and its biological systems are all constantly seeking a state of equilibrium. This mechanism is called *homeostasis* and the movement toward equilibrium is what keeps us in good health.

When our energetic body is balanced, it can readily integrate and correct any information it receives, whatever its nature might be. The planes move, the envelope extends or contracts, and its density or concentration varies. When the source of the influence is no longer active, the energetic body as a whole tries to find its balance once again.

Energetic imbalance takes hold in a permanent way when

a person has been exposed to harmful influences for too long. Homeostasis is disturbed, no longer functions as it should, and areas of blockage settle into the energetic body. These blockages give rise to various illnesses.

How Are Bioenergetic Parameters Detected and Measured?

Each living cell emits an emanation called *mitogenic radiation,* or bioplasma. The ancients, according to their culture, called this emanation *ankh, mana, prana, chi, qi,* or *pneuma.*

This emanation, being extremely weak, is difficult to measure with electronic equipment. Some equipment however manages to capture the interaction of this radiation with matter. Some examples of this are Kirlian photography, GDV bioelectrography (Gas Discharge Visualization), gas chromatography-mass spectrometry, and sensitive crystallization.

Etheric waves are scalar waves, just as thoughts are scalar waves (psychic waves picked up by psychics). The only way to capture them is to use a device that also works with scalar waves: the brain and the chakras. Etheric waves are longitudinal waves that create "packets" of waves locally. In the air, these packets are easily felt with the hands or perceived with the eyes (a sparkling in the air).

Some bioenergetic workers use a pendulum, rods, or antennas to measure energetic emanation. These devices simply amplify the signal perceived by one's own energetic field. In my research, I mainly use my hands as a measuring instrument. Every living being is able to do this. You can teach a child in a few minutes. With adults, you need an average of one or two days for the mind to let go of the belief that energy can't be felt.

Scientific or Unscientific?

In general, modern science applied to our everyday reality is materialistic and is still based on old Newtonian and Darwinian paradigms.

During the twentieth century, the mechanistic view of the world that had dominated physics for almost three hundred years collapsed as we explored the infinitely small and the infinitely large. The new paradigms of quantum physics revolutionized our understanding of matter, space, and time. Our daily life is still partially based on the old paradigms but more and more of us are integrating the new ones by becoming aware of realities that are not totally limited to what we can touch.

Fortunately, the new paradigm is beginning to generate scientific theories such as Rupert Sheldrake's morphogenetic fields and the Akashic fields spoken of by Ervin Laszlo. More and more, these theories indicate a rapprochement between science and a mystical, energetic, and scientific vision of the world that is capable of bridging ancient traditional knowledge and contemporary research.

Many people require scientific guarantees in bioenergetic research. One standard of scientific research is to establish research protocols, apply them, produce results, and verify their reproducibility. This is exactly our procedure in energetic research. Although we measure subtle phenomena easily detectable with our hands, the measurements we take are reproducible. This means that in similar conditions (environmental influences) no matter who is taking the measurements, we obtain similar results. This measuring technique was perfected in 1998 by Swiss architect, geobiologist, and bioenergetic worker Stéphane Cardinaux. Since then, thousands of individuals have been measured in order to draw up complete bioenergetic assessment guidelines. Using these guidelines, Cardinaux has established statistics that have become important benchmarks for all bioenergetic researchers.

I learned these measuring techniques in 2005 and since then I have personally established more than one thousand guidelines designed for therapeutic or teaching purposes. I regularly use these techniques for my bioenergetic research and especially in my research on the effects of minerals and crystals.

RESEARCH ON SHUNGITE

While I am always on the lookout for answers about the effects of the interaction between living things and the emanations of matter, it was by chance that I discovered shungite; the full potential of which I know I have not yet fully explored.

Since passion and reason don't get along well together, we wanted to conduct experiments that would confirm or contradict the very strong felt sense this stone gave us when we held it in our hands for the first time. Therefore, following a rigorous methodology, we carried out double-blind tests in order to assure ourselves that we were not confusing expectations with results.

The double-blind tests were carried out using someone from outside our research group who was unaware of the exact subject of the protocol. Several different minerals, including shungite, were placed in little boxes all of the same size and numbered by an assistant (the numbers were not visible either to the person tested or to the person carrying out the measurements).

A complete bioenergetic assessment was established in the following way:

- Measurement of the vital field in front of the body at three points—high, middle, and low
- Measurement of the vital field behind the body at three points—high, middle, and low
- Measurement of the permeability using the spacing of the sublayers or another technique
- Determining the position of the two principal axes—vertical and horizontal
- Measurement of the emanations from the seven chakras (in front of and behind the body for chakras two through six; above and below the body for chakras one and seven)

The measurements were recorded by a third person who did not know what the boxes contained and used only the box number as the reference. Several minerals were tested during the same session; all of them quite ordinary in their anonymous little boxes. The boxes were shuffled for the next session, and the results were opened and checked once a week.

We worked like that for an initial period of several weeks in order to validate the reliability of our protocol. I must confess that at the end of those few weeks, finding myself surrounded by columns of numbers and boxes, my passion for shungite and crystals began to wane!

However, the first results were convincing. We found identical results for identical stones. We had discovered a good way of validating our overall assessment of the effectiveness of the influence of crystals and minerals on the human bioenergetic system.

Moreover, these first tests confirmed that shungite really was a powerful mineral and that it fulfilled the promise of the energetic and bodily felt sense we had when we simply held a piece of it in our hands.

RESULTS:
THE BIOENERGETIC PROPERTIES
OF SHUNGITE

Let's analyze first of all the following two drawings based on tests carried out on a male subject with an average vital field.

The first test was carried out using an average-sized (10 gram) black shungite (type II) stone. Remember that we examined the different qualities of shungite in "The Different Types of Shungite" in chapter 1. The drawing below shows the vital field and the emanations of the chakras before and after the subject meditated for five minutes with the stone in his hand.* You can see a rather significant increase in the size of the vital field especially in the lower body. This increase took place because of the stimulating action of the shungite, most dramatically on the first chakra which is a great gatherer of energy (as well as the fourth and seventh chakras).

The energy channeled by the first chakra is a dense, concentrated energy that structures and brings the force of life to the whole bioenergetic system. This force, as seen in the drawing, moves out from the base chakra toward all the other higher energetic centers and the length of the emanation of all the chakras increases. Before the meditation with the shungite, we see that the chakras had different lengths; some were shorter

---

*Meditating with a stone consists of being quiet and still for a moment in order to simply connect with the stone that is held in the hand, having no other thoughts, and allowing its energy to circulate freely.

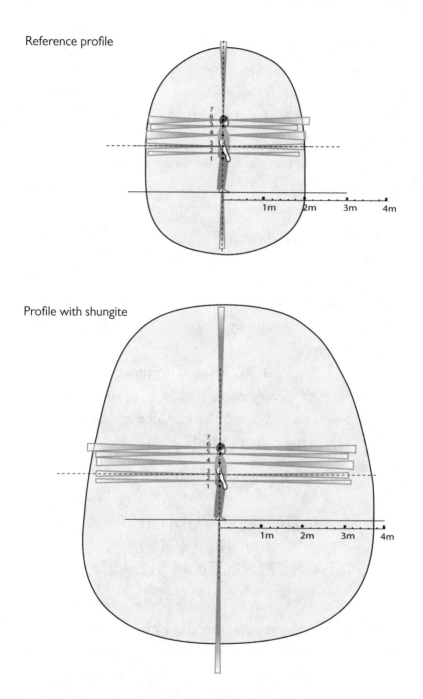

Reference profile

Profile with shungite

Drawing of the effect of a five-minute meditation with a black shungite (type II) stone in the hand.

than the vital field while others extended beyond it based on their greater activation. After the meditation with the black shungite stone, we can see that all the chakras were realigned with each other and with the vital field. This is a sign of balance being restored.

The second test was carried out with a shungite stone of silver quality (type I) of average size (10 grams). We can see in the drawing on the facing page that the increase in size of the vital field is more than in the previous test. The explanation of this phenomenon can be attributed to the fact that silver-quality shungite contains 98 percent carbon and therefore has a proportionately higher quantity of fullerenes. Emanations from all the chakras increase harmoniously. The first and seventh chakras both extend beyond the vital field, which was not the case in the first test. This has the effect of accentuating even more the alignment of the whole energetic body. When the first and seventh chakras extend beyond the envelope of the vital field, they are in very active contact with natural cosmic and telluric emanations.

WHAT DISTINGUISHES SHUNGITE FROM OTHER PROTECTION STONES?

I have carried out detailed studies using bioenergetic tests that were conducted in therapy sessions and I have personally tested more than two hundred stones and crystals that have an influence on one or on a number of chakras. Among those tested, I made comparative studies of about twenty stones, including shungite, that were able to resonate with the first chakra.

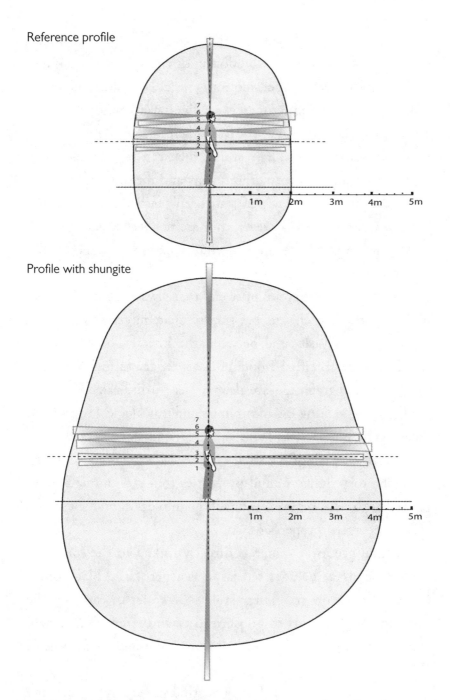

Reference profile

Profile with shungite

1m 2m 3m 4m 5m

Drawing of the effect of a five-minute meditation with a silver shungite (type I) stone in the hand.

Some of them are quite powerful including black obsidian, galena, black tourmaline, labradorite, turritella agate, black tektite, spectrolite, iron jasper, morion quartz, cerussite, and anglesite. They vibrate and resonate with the lower part of the body, specifically with the area of the feet. Their low vibration substantially concentrates us. These stones then can be very useful in certain ways for initiatory lithotherapy and for sessions of meditation that are designed to penetrate deeply buried and sometimes blocked information. However, they are not recommended for a daily practice linked to life and vitality except for expert, fully informed users.

There is another group of stones that always act on the emanations of the first chakra, but they resonate more with a chakra outside the body situated between the knees. These stones—which include silicified wood, chiastolite, crystalline hematite, magnetite, and graphite—are also very useful and valued for deep work and for looking into our family and genealogical roots from an energetic perspective.

Of course, each of the stones in the two groups above has its own vibratory signature and properties that are unique to that particular stone. This book is unable go into detail on each stone's specific energetic properties.

A final group of minerals directly linked to the source of the first chakra includes red jasper, garnet, flint, black onyx, jet, and smoky quartz. These stones are easier to carry on the body for long periods to boost vitality and strength and help the wearer to be more grounded. I place shungite right here in this group.

In comparing tests on shungite with tests carried out on other stones of this group, we noticed right away that among stones of the same weight, shungite achieves the largest expansion of the vital field, the greatest concentration, and a strikingly significant expansion of the first chakra. The other significant finding was that the balance among the other chakras was not disturbed in spite of the increase in concentration and extent of the first chakra's field. This characteristic of shungite is much less present in other stones of the first group.

Once the strength of shungite had been verified on a balanced energetic body in a neutral state, I moved on to a subsequent stage in order to find out for myself if the experiments carried out in Russia pertaining to health, left torsion fields, and electromagnetic waves were verifiable using the techniques of bioenergy.

We had to be able to prove that shungite acted on the energetic system as a protector and transformer of electromagnetic waves. A series of tests were conducted and a brochure containing the results was published in 2008 in order to help users choose solutions adapted to their needs. A core part of this research is found in appendix 1 at the end of this book. A small series of tests were also conducted by Stéphane Cardinaux using the bioelectrographic procedure of GDV capture (Kirlian technique). These tests are described in appendix 2.

It is quite possible that the presence of fullerenes would explain all of shungite's qualities:

1. The property of helping the energetic body instantaneously correct the influence of left torsion fields
2. The property of neutralizing the impact of electromagnetic radiation
3. The ability to open access to life energy (first chakra)

4. The ability to concentrate the vital field
5. The property of not taking on negative charges

1. Instantaneous Correction of the Influence of Left Torsion Fields

At every moment, our energetic body is continuously informed and influenced by everything around it. It picks up and integrates subtle information from everything that it comes into contact with, whether we're aware of it or not. As we saw above, the influence of left torsion fields, which are created from everything that is artificial, shifts our vertical axis and totally unbalances our bioenergetic system. This system tries to rebalance itself every moment, but if the influence is present for long periods it can permanently upset the energetic system and disturb it to the point where it influences the physical plane, giving rise to dysfunction and illness.

When shungite is in direct contact with the physical body or when it is present as a nearby emanation (see the action of spheres or pyramids of shungite in chapter 7, "Practical Applications"), it helps the energetic body instantaneously correct the shifting of the plane to the left and allows the system as a whole to remain centered. It also allows the individual to be connected to telluric energy and cosmic energy in a natural and positive way. This ability is what is commonly called *protection*.

This property of shungite is its main asset. This is what makes it a stone of protection and also a stone that accompanies the healing of a number of illnesses.

2. Neutralizing the Impact of Electromagnetic Radiation

Another of shungite's great assets, which mainly accounts for its recent fame, is its ability to protect us from electromagnetic radiation.

This radiation is one of the principal sources of left torsion fields. They are very harmful to our health and especially detrimental to our overall energetic balance, which includes all of the following levels: physical, energetic, emotional, psychic, and spiritual.

The rapid technological development of our society has brought us into contact all day long with a large quantity of these sources of harmful radiation, and very often we are quite unaware this is happening. It is clear that we need to find solutions so that humankind can survive its own technology.

For about fifteen years, a number of researchers in the field of bioenergy have endeavored to identify systems that would allow individuals to reestablish their equilibrium. However, it has only been recently that the public at large is beginning to be more fully informed about the health problems created by the increase in electromagnetic radiation. A simple, efficient, inexpensive solution is what we need—shungite.

Our research on shungite demonstrated its effectiveness in neutralizing the effects of electric fields, electromagnetic fields, and pulsed electromagnetic fields such as those emitted by home appliances, cordless phones (DECT), cell phones, Wi-Fi hot spots, and computers—in short, all of the electromagnetic emissions that generally surround us.

We conducted two kinds of experiments: one was to test the different ways the impact of electromagnetic fields on the individual could be corrected and the other was to try to correct the harmful information directly at its source. In both cases we obtained totally satisfying results with shungite. A complete account of these tests is provided in appendix 1.

It would be useful to make an important comment on the "correcting" of the emanations from electromagnetic fields to avoid any possible misunderstanding. The transformative effect of shungite appears essentially at the bioenergetic level: one could say that it transforms a left torsion influence into a right torsion influence.

Although electromagnetic waves are invisible, they have a physical component and it is this physical component that is picked up by the commonly used electromagnetic field detectors. When the influence is modified on a subtler energetic level, the physical emanation is still picked up by the detection equipment. In other words, the shungite does not interfere with the functioning of this equipment. It doesn't turn off the pulsed waves emitted by a Wi-Fi transmitter, a cordless phone, or a cell phone. Instead it transforms the influence of harmful radiation. It is quite clear that the solution is not to eliminate the radiation but instead to prevent its deleterious impact on our health.

This especially important property of shungite can be illustrated with an example drawn from an experiment carried out recently in Russia. Researchers went to a site where poultry was being raised and for twenty-one days they studied three incubators, each of which contained ninety-eight hen's eggs. They placed a cell phone in standby mode in the center of the first incubator. The second incubator contained another cell phone in standby mode, positioned on a shungite plate. The third incubator was the control and was used in the normal way. At the end of twenty-one days, the control group had a loss rate of 11.2 percent. The incubator with an unprotected portable phone had only twenty-one chicks hatched—a loss rate of 79.42 percent! The incubator with the cell phone that had shungite protection came in with a loss rate of 10.5 percent. The figures speak for themselves.

A similar experiment was conducted in France by researchers at the Immunology and Parasitology Laboratory of the University of Montpellier, but they didn't use shungite. Only the harmful effects of the electromagnetic waves from cell phones (without protection) were measured in the incubators. The results of the measurement of harmful effects were about the same as those in the Russian experiment.

3. Opening Access to Life Energy (First Chakra)

Our vital energy results from a subtle cosmic and telluric alchemy that our body activates between the concentrated, dense energy of the Earth (telluric energy) and cosmic energies.

The two main entryways for these energies are as follows: for the cosmic energy, the seventh chakra or crown chakra, which is found at the top of the head (fontanelle); and for the telluric energy, the first chakra, which is situated in the lower part of the body (perineum).

The majority of crystals that have enjoyed great success with the public—such as amethyst, rock crystal, and fluorite—have a very high vibration and connect us to the most subtle planes (spiritual planes) allowing us to connect easily with cosmic energy through the upper chakras. These crystals dilate the vital field, but at the same time its concentration decreases. In order to come back to an energetic balance, it is essential to also come to a harmony between higher and lower.

What we call *anchoring, rootedness,* or *grounding* is a natural function of our energetic body; it involves the first chakra, which is radiating downward toward the ground. We are connected to the Earth through the first chakra; it's what keeps us alive and in the present moment. The density or concentration of matter, of our physical body, of our strength, of our endurance, and of our vitality depends on the quality of our link with the Earth and on the emanation and opening of the first chakra.

Shungite helps us return to the naturalness of this contact and to connect us once again to the energy of life. In experiencing shungite, we can instinctively feel the strength of this contact in our whole body, as if all the cells were becoming entrained in a unique dance, the dance of life.

4. Concentrating the Vital Field

Another basic element of the effects of shungite is to be found in the great increase in the concentration of the vital field. This is one of the reasons that this stone is a so-called protection stone. When we feel weakened, or feel that our strength is depleted, it means that our energetic concentration is low, making us more vulnerable to influences from our environment.

The concentration or density is directly linked to the strength or to the emanation distance of the first chakra; that is, to the anchoring. In my training sessions and workshops I prefer to use the word *rootedness*. The word *anchoring* refers to the anchor we cast in order to stabilize a boat that, without it, would be carried away by the current. It more or less implies that our first chakra was a last hope thrown to the earth so we are not swept away. The image is very evocative, and probably not inaccurate for certain individuals, but I prefer to highlight an alternate symbolism.

Rootedness makes us think of a tree that develops roots before sending out its branches and leaves toward the sky. Without roots a tree cannot enjoy a full realization of its potential. In just the same way, we as human beings have an imperative necessity for our stability, our vital force, and our awareness of reality to be present. And this takes place with our feet on the ground and our subtle roots welcoming and being nourished by the Earth's energy.

Bioenergetic concentration or density makes up a large part of our protection. If, for example, we look carefully at all the lithotherapy stones described as being protection stones, we see that mostly these are stones that increase the concentration of the vital field and activate the first chakra. The concentration of the vital field, and consequently the reinforcement of our bioenergetic system, happens through the first chakra and shows up as an increase in the number of sublayers of the vital field as well as an increase in the emanations of the first chakra.

The practical consequence of this concentration is a greater resistance to external disturbances and an enhanced capacity to recover from illnesses or from emotional shocks. This concentration is a characteristic of the protection effect of all stones that activate rootedness (of which shungite is one of the representative stones).

Because of the presence of fullerenes in its composition, shungite has an additional property of activating energetic circulation.

5. Not Taking on Negative Charges

It is likely because of the presence of fullerenes that shungite does not take on a charge when exposed to sources such as electromagnetic radiation, high frequencies, or human emotional influences.

The empty interior of the natural fullerene molecules present in shungite (hollow geodesic molecules) creates a microvortex of dextrorotatory energy that keeps all the properties mentioned above in an active state.

All matter existing in the universe is also vibration and movement. Shungite is one of those substances that emits a maximum of right torsion fields. It is this characteristic that allows shungite to offer more resistance to the impact of left torsion fields and to transform them into right torsion fields.

7

PRACTICAL
APPLICATIONS

Here we are finally at the point of discussing how we can use this exceptional stone in our lives. Having a large quantity of shungite artifacts available, as well as simple unworked stones, polished black shungite, and silver shungite, is a situation we expect will continue. I'm going to speak about all these forms; each with its own specific nature and utility.

First of all, in order to appreciate the energetic quality of shungite, you can simply get yourself a polished stone that you hold in your hand or keep with you in your bag or in your pocket. Also, you can hold a piece of silver-quality shungite in your hand and appreciate its energetic message. Take a silent moment for yourself or do a short meditation and try to listen to what is taking place within as you hold a piece of shungite. Do not be the least bit upset, however, if you don't feel anything in particular because shungite will have its effect in any case. Our tests have confirmed that the influence of shungite on the bioenergetic parameters is the same for two individuals having the same stone in their hands, even if one of them feels the energy and the other does not. So, have confidence. It doesn't take any particular gift to be able to feel—only a bit of patience to come back to a natural felt sense.

My experience in leading workshops in lithotherapy and bioenergy has shown me that anyone who takes a little time will manage sooner or later to feel the internal movements of energy and will be able to measure energy fields. Regaining one's spontaneous capacity to feel contributes to a sense of fullness and to a connection with what is natural. Shungite, which is a stone of life energy, can guide us and open for us a path of self-discovery.

SHAPE CHARACTERISTICS

The forms we speak about below are worked in black shungite which can vary in purity depending on the presence of differing numbers of veins of pyrite or silica, as well as the quantities of imperfections and inclusions.

Pyramids

Pyramids are, in general, very much appreciated for the beauty of their form and for the power they release. (See plate 6 of the color insert for a photo of shungite pyramids.) A pyramid emits its own form waves* that carry the shungite influence quite a distance. For example, a pyramid with a 7 cm (2.8 inch) high side emanates

---

*A form wave is a subtle emanation of matter. Each object emits an emanation that corresponds to its form and to its vibration (vibratory signature).

perceptibly (in a neutral area) up to 3 meters (9.8 feet) from its flat side or 3.4 meters (11 feet) from each of its edges.

Spheres

Spheres emit a more uniform and harmonious emanation and are ideal for living rooms and bedrooms. (See plate 7.) A sphere with a diameter of 6 cm (2.4 inches) emanates perceptibly up to 3.4 meters (11 feet). Spheres have a harmonizing power over our energetic body because this form is in resonance with the shape of our vital field.

Small spheres of shungite are often used for relaxation and meditation, or paired with other stones as harmonizers.

Cubes

Cubes are also often used. (See plate 8.) Their form is in resonance with the Earth and with the first chakra, which reinforces shungite's action of rootedness. Their power is said to be less than the two preceding forms. In fact, a cube with sides of 6 cm (2.4 inches), even when it contains more shungite and is therefore heavier than a sphere with a diameter of 6 cm (2.4 inches), emits only to a distance of 2.9 meters (9.5 feet).

Eggs

A symbol of origins used by almost all peoples of the Earth in their cosmologies and the perfect form of alchemists, the egg harmonizes the space around it. (See plate 9.)

It emanates a wave of agreeable form that connects us more to life in all of its forms, both physical and spiritual. An egg of 150 grams (5.3 ounces) can emanate up to 3 meters (9.8 feet).

SHUNGITE AS ELECTROMAGNETIC PROTECTION

The choice of protection can be divided into two distinct systems: either wearing or carrying the protection or changing the signal emitted by the apparatus using a localized protection.

In the first case, we are modifying the parameters of our own energetic system by using a stone that increases its concentration or density through reinforcing the first chakra. This method allows our bioenergetic system to continuously correct the harmful interference.

In the second case, we apply the protective influence to the harmful source and this corrects and transforms the electromagnetic waves into biocompatible emanations. In the case of pulsed electromagnetic waves (Wi-Fi, cordless phones, and cell phones) the corrected influence emanates with the same strength as the original, harmful source but in a biocompatible and positive way.

About Harmful Sources

As we have already seen, modifying the influence of electromagnetic radiation is something shungite knows how to do very well, and much better than other stones because shungite does not become saturated, does not take on a negative charge, and powerfully keeps on transforming the radiation into biocompatible elements (right torsion fields). Detailed information on the shungite tests with radiation can be found in appendix 1.

For example, if we use a detection device to measure the emission field of a Wi-Fi hot spot protected with a shungite plate, we will quite happily still find the Wi-Fi signal doing its job of connecting two devices wirelessly with its waves. What changes and what is not revealed by the detection device is the subtle quality of the emanation, the biocompatibility of the waves with your energy when there is a shungite plate, and the fact that the emanation is negative when the plate is not there.

There are many forms of shungite that can be used with equipment that emits harmful radiation. The following recommendations apply in the same proportions to any electromagnetic equipment that you have to use or want to use.

Cell Phones

As an initial step, I recommend the protection of cell phones because you only need a small adhesive disc or a pendant that you wear in order to completely neutralize the harmful effects of these waves, which attack your energetic balance, your health, and especially, given the way cell phones are held, your cerebral and auditory functions.

Wi-Fi Hot Spots

I receive a lot of questions and requests for advice about Wi-Fi, and especially about Wi-Fi from your neighbors, because very often when you start up your computer and you take a look at the number of Wi-Fi signals present in your home (in a city this can amount to eight, ten, or even fifteen), you can get upset just seeing the number of all these signals. Carrying a shungite stone on one's person or placing shungite objects in your home can provide protection from Wi-Fi signals that are coming from your neighbors.

In order to transform the radiations from your own Wi-Fi hot spot, transmitter, or router, we recommend placing the transmission base on a large plate of polished shungite, or even attaching the plate to the side of the transmitter (using adhesive stickers). In order to ensure an effective transformation of the emanations, you need to use a polished stone of type II shungite weighing a minimum of 10 to 15 grams (0.4 to 0.5 ounce), or a piece of silver quality shungite of at least 10 grams (0.4 ounce). There are round plates designed for computers that can also be used with a Wi-Fi base.

Laptops

Laptop computers, which are also widely used, are harmful as well. This is not so much because of the screen, which does not radiate negatively the way the old cathode-ray screens used to do, but more because of the hard drive's motor and its active components. We advise placing a round plate or stone on the computer beside the keyboard. The action of the shungite will bring relief to the user, particularly when using the keyboard and the mouse. In order to benefit from a stronger effect and to combat the fatigue that accompanies working on a laptop, the effect of the shungite plate can be enhanced by also having a shungite stone in one's pocket or wearing it as a pendant.

For those who spend many hours in front of a computer screen, the most comprehensive protection is a shungite cushion. Sitting on a cushion containing 1 kg (2.2 lbs) of shungite allows you to benefit from its activating effect the entire time you are seated.

Cordless Phones

Something many people are less aware of is that often we have a very harmful source of radiation in our homes—the cordless phone. The base of a cordless phone in fact emits harmful bioenergetic waves that extend out all around it to a distance of around 10 meters (33 feet). You can check out the diagrams in appendix 1 to learn more about the damaging effects.

Since the radiation has its source in the base of the phone, it is essential to protect the base (or to opt for a nonportable phone). Once the information from the base has been positively transformed by the shungite, each connected handset automatically emits right torsion fields instead of left torsion fields. Torsion fields are transmitted by the electromagnetic waves.

In correcting the negative influence from the bases of cordless phones, we recommend a shungite plate, or a shungite stone of a minimum of 15 grams (0.5 ounce) for black polished shungite and a minimum of 10 grams (0.4 ounce) for silver shungite.

Electrical Panels

It is useful to place a shungite pyramid on the electrical distribution panel of a house or apartment. Having it there will correct the damaging influence of 60 Hz alternating current that is typically emitted by electrical installations in the United States. For a studio or small apartment, a pyramid of 5 cm (2 inches) is enough. The more extensive the electric installation, the larger the pyramid should be. For a house without electric heating, a pyramid of 7 cm (2.8 inches) is likely enough.

Microwaves

Microwave ovens are a touchy topic, as this equipment is a basic tool among our electric appliances. It is so commonly used that we tend to pay little attention to how it works. For many people, the microwave oven is completely harmless. For some people, you need only protect yourself from residual waves (such as poor seals on the door) by positioning shungite there or using other handy means of protection. But then, what good does it do to protect yourself externally from a device that destroys and irradiates what you ingest moments later? A microwave oven uses microwaves to excite the molecules of water that are present in our food in order to heat it. The bioenergetic measurements taken by all practitioners show that all food and drink that is cooked or heated in microwave ovens, causes us to lose from 40 percent to 60 percent of our vital field following its ingestion.

The only possible protection, in bioenergetic terms, is *never* to use them and therefore to not even have a microwave oven in the home. If you value your health, stop using them. It's as simple as that.

Carrying or Wearing Shungite

Another way of protecting yourself from the electromagnetic waves that now assail our lives from all sides consists of carrying or wearing shungite on the body.

As has been explained in the preceding chapters, shungite acts on our energetic body as a concentrator and an activator; transforming in real time the impact of left torsion fields on our vital systems.

There are various workplace situations (offices, factories, businesses) where many people have to share space with several others. In such cases you can't necessarily act directly on the sources of the harmful radiation and people who are aware of the harmful nature of the waves, surrounded by others who are not, have no other option except to transform their own energy.

Nowadays, there is a wide selection of pendants of all shapes that can be worn as jewelry or more discretely under one's clothing. Sometimes it only takes a few grams of shungite worn against the skin to feel the concentrating and activating effect. Some pendants are in polished black shungite and others are in silver shungite, which can be smaller but which have a much stronger effect.

For even greater protection, depending on the requirements of the external circumstances or on hypersensitivity, there are necklaces or bracelets that have very powerful and effective pearls of shungite. However, they should not be worn for too long, at least not at the beginning, because for people in good shape they can produce a surfeit of energy. In contrast however, necklaces or bracelets are excellent for the rehabilitation of weakened or convalescent individuals.

Shungite and Locales

If you detect a general problematic situation connected to electromagnetic emissions in a place you often frequent, such as your home or place of work, and it is impossible for you to intervene directly at the source of these emissions, you can nevertheless intervene by placing shungite at carefully chosen strategic points in that locale.

Here are a few concrete examples.

Say you have a relay tower transmitting in the direction of your apartment and you feel the effects of it in symptoms of exhaustion, fatigue, insomnia, extreme nervousness, or irritability. What you need to do then is to place remedial objects in areas where you spend the most time—for example, in the living room you can place a large pyramid of shungite with sides of 7 or 8 cm (about 3 inches) or more depending on the size of the room. For a bedroom you have to be a little more careful—simply placing a shungite sphere or egg on the bedside table. However, while shungite protects against the wave pollution, it can provide too much vital energy and prevent you from falling asleep, so for light sleepers I recommend using alchemical pairs of eggs and spheres to balance the information given to your energetic body during the night. Pairing up eggs and spheres—one of shungite and one of selenite—is perfect for peaceful nights. The shungite eliminates the radiation of left torsion fields and selenite provides deep relaxation and letting go, which facilitates sleep.

In the case of living quarters that are near high-tension lines, the best thing would be to move elsewhere. However, shungite can help to lessen the damaging effects of high-tension electric lines on your health. You can wear a shungite pendant during the day and protect each room of the home using a large pyramid of 8 or 9 cm (about 3.5 inches) or a sphere with a minimum diameter of 6 cm (2.4 inches).

For those who feel the influence of Wi-Fi or cordless phones in their home or coming from neighbors, we also advise shungite objects (pyramids, spheres, eggs) in every room. However, they can be smaller than what is advised in the case of more serious structural influences (such as high-tension electric transmission lines).

Oftentimes in a single office that has a concentration of several electromagnetic wave sources, using a large pyramid of at least 7 cm (2.8 inches) can resolve the problem. However, you have to remember that pyramids and other shungite objects come in certain dimensions and have a corresponding effect on the space around them that depends on their size. As soon as you leave that space, the pulsed waves from Wi-Fi or cordless phones return with most of their negative vibrational effects. If you have a home office, you may often forget to turn off one or more pieces of equipment that generate pulsed electromagnetic waves, and just placing a pyramid or some other object in the office is not going to be enough to entirely protect the space beyond that room. So if your bedroom is beyond the area that is protected, there will likely be disturbed sleep due to the pulsed waves. That's why it is preferable to protect the Wi-Fi or cordless phone base at its source using shungite which will transform the nature of the pulsed waves no matter how far you are away from their source.

If however it's a case of electrosensitivity in general, you should go to appendix 3 of this book to look into this problem more deeply.

SHUNGITE FOR WELL-BEING

All the Russian studies on using shungite for therapeutic purposes have demonstrated its effectiveness and its ability in stimulating immune system defenses and in reactivating healing processes (see chapter 5 on Russian research relating to this topic).

From our nonmedical point of view, we are interested in applying shungite to the domain of well-being. In its natural state and in whatever form it may be, this mineral displays no negative effect whatever. It is therefore ideal for usage without precise therapeutic control. However, as with any solution linked to well-being, the use of shungite never replaces the advice of a medical doctor when faced with any specific pathology.

The advantage to the use of shungite is that it is never in conflict with other therapies, even those that depend on medication, because it acts on the base of our energetic body and supports all efforts taken to reestablish balance and health.

Drinking Shungite Water

The first historically recognized use of shungite was that of spring water gushing up from shungite rocks in the region around Lake Onega in Karelia. It was by drinking this water that the inhabitants of the region became aware of its properties. The use of this water over the centuries is living proof of the well-being that it brought to the population and its consumption is more than ever of current relevance.

Of course importing spring water would be costly and complicated because it would mean creating infrastructures that don't exist in Karelia. However, shungite properties manifest easily just by putting raw black shungite pebbles in contact with drinking water.

As we all know, tap water coming from domestic water supplies is disinfected with chlorine and other chemical products. Constantly using this water for drinking and cooking without any additional purification means that our bodies are permanently in contact with these molecules even if there are only traces of them remaining.

In addition, tap water is repeatedly subjected to pumping through powerful electric pumps, which generate intense electromagnetic fields. This completely destroys the living structure of the water. Consequently, we get tap water that is "dead water" with its structure broken. Imbibing this water has a negative impact on the cells of our body and on the proteins, and it augments the proliferation of free radicals, which contributes to cellular aging.

The filters that are currently used partially remove pollutants but they do not restore the water's natural dynamic quality.

With its power to reactivate and revitalize, shungite gives

water back its ability to hydrate our tissues and penetrate deeply into cellular structures.

Shungite water can be regularly used as an energizing drink. (See plate 10 of the color insert.) If you are in good health, we advise drinking a glass every morning (but take a week-long break from it once a month). If you are sick or convalescent, you could drink 2 or 3 glasses a day. Shungite water has no secondary effects. Like all regenerative and purifying food and drink, it can stimulate the draining of toxins from the body and thereby speed up processes that are underway. Also, as with all energizing drinks, consuming shungite water is not recommended in large doses.

How to Prepare Shungite Water

Wash shungite pebbles by rubbing them with your hands or using a brush to remove any fine black powder.

Place about 100 grams (3.5 ounces) of shungite pebbles per liter (2.1 pints) of water at the bottom of a glass or ceramic carafe.

Leave the shungite in this water for three days in order to obtain maximum effect. Then your activated water will be ready to drink. Begin the process over again, continuing to refill your container regularly.

Shungite keeps indefinitely. There is no risk of it getting negatively charged. However, in order to keep this preparation physically clean (avoiding an accumulation of nitrates, chlorine, and so forth), we advise purifying the pebbles in the sun every four to six months. If the water you use is heavily chlorinated or polluted, we recommend changing the pebbles every two or three years.

You can also place shungite pebbles on the bottom of a carafe fitted with a filter. The water is already filtered and the shungite can more readily deploy its activating power. This also works well with osmosis-processed water, which is very pure but if it is missing vital and dynamic qualities shungite can put that back in the water.

Shungite water can be used in compresses or when washing as daily maintenance to maintain the elasticity and tone of the skin. Shungite's fullerenes speed up the skin regeneration process and because of that it can help with juvenile acne and other skin problems.

Shungite Baths

Baths in water containing shungite can be very useful in regaining energy and well-being, reducing fatigue, and improving circulation. In order to prepare a shungite bath, shungite pebbles are placed in a sachet bag that is left in the bath for ten minutes.

For maximum effect, you need to remain in the bath for about twenty minutes.

Wearing Shungite: Pendants, Jewelry, and Belts

Wearing a beautiful stone is a pleasure. The first instinct of someone who loves crystals is to slip a stone into a pocket. Not a bad idea; but do it with awareness because forgetting about a stone that gets lost in a jacket pocket with car keys and tissues is likely to have a less than optimal influence.

Having a piece of shungite on one's person, as we have seen earlier, protects, tones, and adds vitality. When you're a little tired, all you need to do is hold the stone in your hand for three minutes and, by "contacting" it, your vital energy will return instantly.

Having a shungite stone handy can be quite useful in small, daily emergencies. For example, in the case of a small burn or cut, place a piece of shungite on the affected area and let it work there for about ten minutes. Healing will take place more quickly because the shungite activates localized, self-healing power by speeding up reaction processes in the body tissues.

Something else you can do is to place two polished type II black shungite stones or two discs of shungite on your closed eyelids as you stretch out for a few minutes. This really helps eye strain after a day of work especially when it was mostly in front of a computer screen.

Wearing a pendant at the level of the heart chakra brings the stone into contact with a very receptive point and increases its beneficial effect.

A necklace of shungite pearls, because of its size, will exercise a powerful effect on the whole energetic body.

Bracelets are also very effective because the wrist is traversed by many meridian lines. They are especially useful for those people who are in contact with a computer mouse or a telephone all day. Bracelets can ward off numbness in the arm.

Earrings, although they are small in size, are useful in protecting the ear from the impact of waves coming from cell phones or cordless phones.

You can also find cloth belts filled with shungite pebbles that can be worn around the waist or on painful or depleted areas. During convalescence they are very effective in restoring lost vitality to the whole body as well as during periods of sustained effort.

Although such belts are very effective and invigorating, they are temporary measures and should not be used every day. If you begin wearing a belt, try it first for a few hours and then increase its use by stages. Listen to your body—it knows its own needs and will be able to tell you when you don't need to wear the belt any more.

The Harmonizers

We use the term *harmonizers* for two identical stone shapes of different composition that are used together. They can be in the shape of cylinders, spheres, or eggs. They are sometimes designed as complementary, instead of identical, paired forms such as a circle and a triangle.

This tradition of paired harmonizers comes from ancient Egypt. The pharaohs are often represented holding a cylinder in each hand while surrounded by two divinities symbolizing *ba* and *ka* energy polarities. For the ancient Egyptians, ba and ka were the two constituent elements of human nature, the two sources of essential, vital energy. The ka cylinder held in the right hand symbolizes the flow of solar energy (masculine principle). The ba cylinder held in the left hand represents the flow of lunar energy (female principle).

The cylinder of the moon acts as a catalyzer, reinforcing the activity of the solar cylinder. In our context, the catalyzing cylinder (yin or lunar) is made of shungite and the other is shaped from other stones chosen for their solar or yang properties. Harmonizers work on the principle of a "difference in potential" between the two stones. A current of subtle energy runs through the body of the person holding the cylinders. The type of energizing and rebalancing effect of this energetic flow is related to the specific qualities of the different stones used.

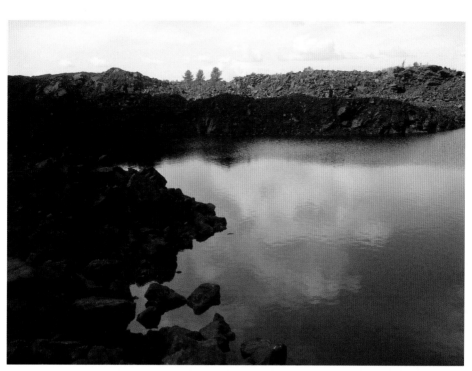

Plate 1. A shungite mine

Plate 2. Type I shungite showing a silvery shine

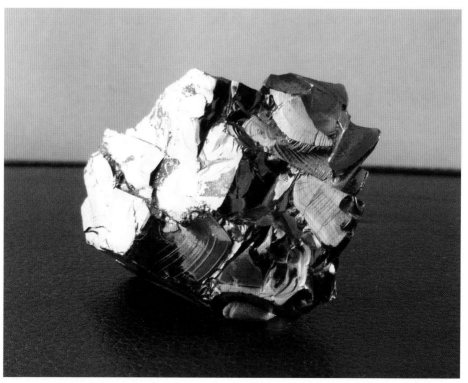

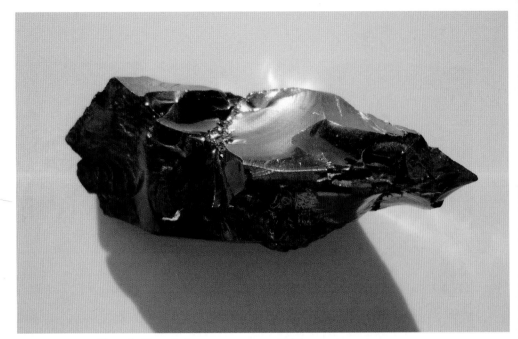

Plate 3. Type I shungite contains 98% organic carbon.

Plate 4. Another example of type I shungite. Type I accounts for only 1% of all shungite that is found.

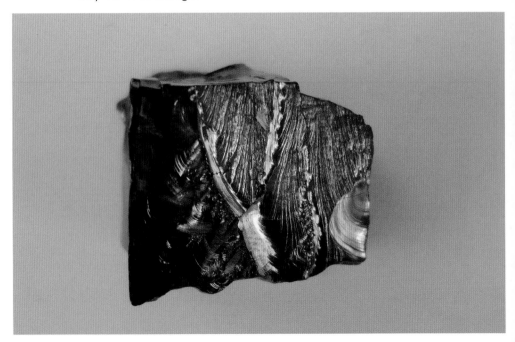

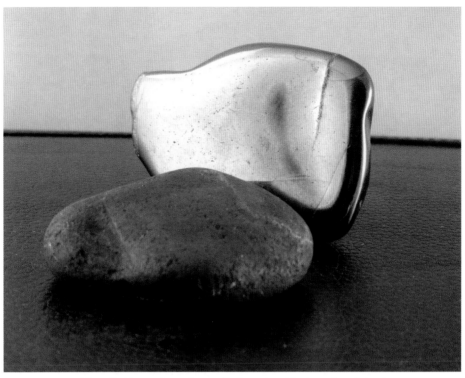

Plate 5. Examples of type II shungite, black and polished

Plate 6. Shungite pyramids emit waveforms that carry the shungite influence quite a distance.

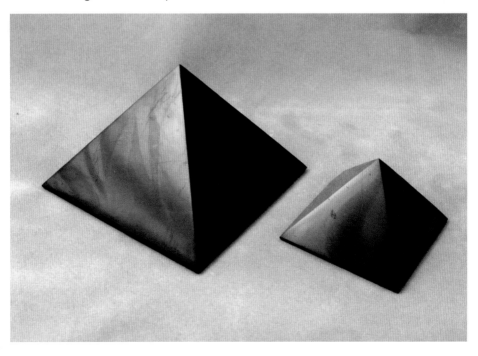

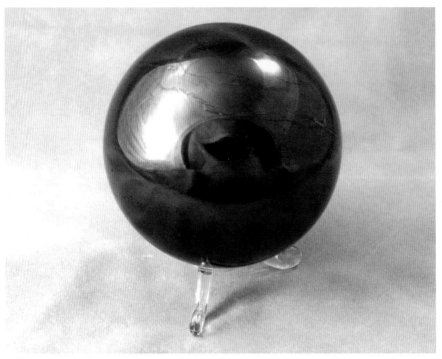

Plate 7. The harmonious emanations of shungite spheres make them ideal for placement in living rooms and bedrooms.

Plate 8. A gray shungite cube. Cubes resonate with the Earth and with the first chakra, reinforcing shungite's action of rootedness.

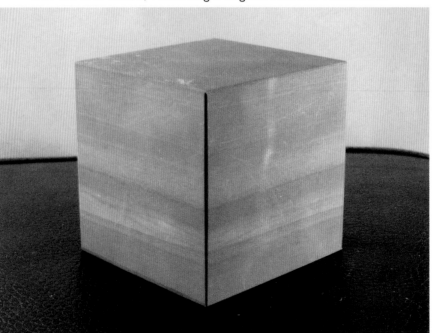

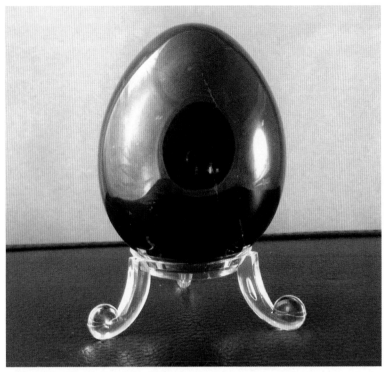

Plate 9. Shungite eggs harmonize the surrounding space and enhance connections among all life-forms.

Plate 10. A carafe of shungite water

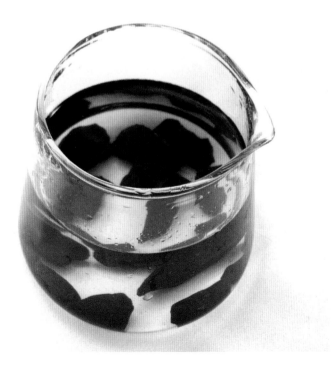

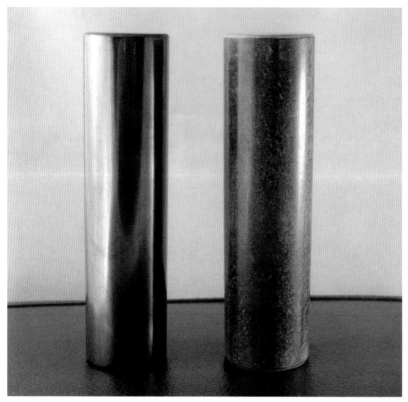

Plate 11. Harmonizer cylinders, shungite (left) and steatite (right)

Plate 12. Crushed shungite used for agricultural purposes. Shungite can absorb and neutralize harmful chemicals and support balance.

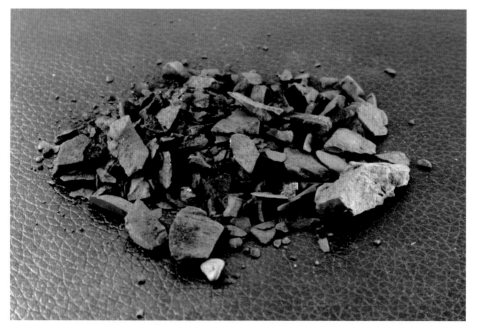

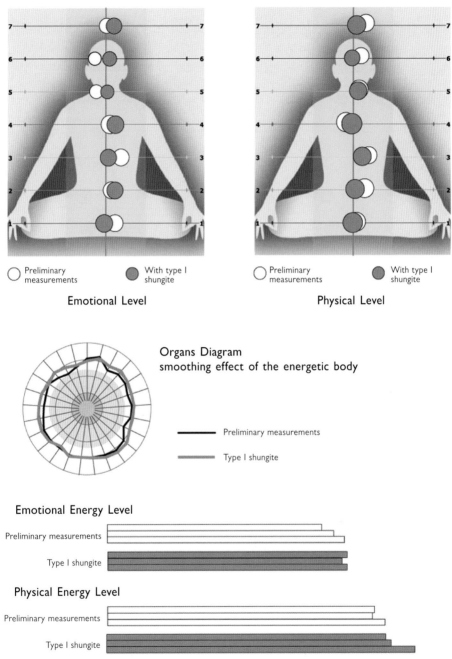

Chakra Measurements

Emotional Level

○ Preliminary measurements ● With type I shungite

Physical Level

○ Preliminary measurements ● With type I shungite

Organs Diagram
smoothing effect of the energetic body

—— Preliminary measurements
—— Type I shungite

Emotional Energy Level
Preliminary measurements
Type I shungite

Physical Energy Level
Preliminary measurements
Type I shungite

Plate 13. Bioelectrographic GDV test results for type I shungite

Testing for Protection against Electromagnetic Fields

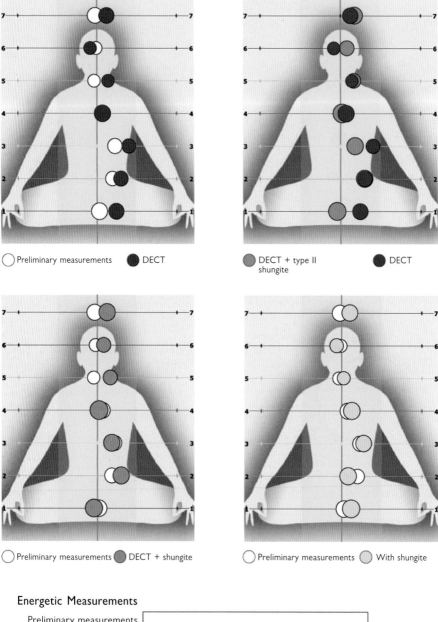

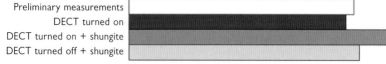

Plate 14. Bioelectrographic GDV test results for type II shungite

The harmonizers created in Russia that you most often find are made of shungite and Karelian steatite. (See plate 11 of the color insert for a photo of a pair of these harmonizers.) Steatite (soapstone) is a soft, gray stone that vibrates with the upper part of the energetic body and supports a good active exchange with shungite, which stimulates the lower part of the body. There are cylinders, spheres, and other shapes carved from these two minerals and originating from the same region.

We also find other combinations of stones paired with shungite. The following is not an exhaustive list:

Seraphinite and Shungite Cylinders

Seraphinite is a very beautiful stone from Siberia, dark green in color with silver white plumes (like the feathers in seraph wings) giving it its strong vibration. Seraphinite, which is known scientifically as clinochlore, connects information from higher levels to the heart chakra.

This pair of harmonizing cylinders brings together the powerful anchoring and energetic purification of shungite with the vibratory power of seraphinite. This aids in the development of extrasensory gifts while amplifying the energetic body and the back of the sixth chakra (intuition area). Shungite supports the anchoring of subtle information which we receive thanks to the development of our extrasensory abilities.

Charoite and Shungite Cylinders

Charoite also comes from Russia. It was named after the Chara River where it was discovered in 1947. It was only in 1978 that it was given a mineralogical name. It is violet in color ranging through various tonalities from light to dark and has white striations and black inclusions.

Charoite opens the energetic body to subtle messages from the high violet vibratory range.

This pair of harmonizing cylinders brings together the powerful anchoring and energetic purification of shungite with the intense vibratory activation of the seventh chakra from the charoite. The work on these two chakras makes this pair perfect for balancing polarities so as to move toward a total alignment of energies.

Nephrite Jade and Shungite Cylinders

Nephrite jade has been known for thousands of years for its curative properties, especially in Asia. The name *nephrite,* which distinguishes it from Burmese jadeite, refers to the use of the stone by the Chinese to treat energetic pathologies of the kidneys.

This pair of harmonizing cylinders brings together the powerful anchoring and energetic purification of shungite with jade's quality of restoring our ability to integrate ancestral memory. This extraordinary combination of two cylinders allows us to contact, treat, and eliminate negative stagnation in the emotions in the lower part of the energetic body (from the diaphragm to the perineum and from the fourth to the seventh chakra).

How to Use Harmonizers

As with all advice in lithotherapy, nothing can replace personal experience—dosages and application times will vary for each one of us.

However, here is a method to begin with:

- Take a seated position but keep very straight without crossing the legs (if you are on a chair) or on a cushion with the legs crossed.
- Hold the shungite cylinder in the left hand and the other stone cylinder in the right hand.
- Put your hands against your thighs keeping the cylinders in a vertical position.
- Close your eyes.
- Concentrate on the physical sensations, become aware of your breathing for a few moments in order to calm your thoughts, then observe and sense the energetic flow that is moving through your body.

Begin with short sessions of three or four minutes, increasing them to ten or fifteen minutes.

It can be interesting to experiment with changing the polarity, holding the shungite cylinder in the right hand and the other cylinder in the left hand for a few minutes. You can also conduct meditations based on these changes in polarity by alternating the position of the cylinders twice in a single session.

In order that the reharmonization and activation of energy is correctly stimulated, we advise using the harmonizers for one or two sessions a day (two sessions if it is clear that there is a state of unbalance) for three weeks, then discontinuing it for a week. As in all things, it is important not to overdo it in energetic practices by engaging in continual stimulation. Always factor in time for a break.

Using harmonizers, you can sense a large energetic flow in the body, moving up in a spiral from below. Some people experience higher states of consciousness and an activation of extrasensory abilities.

If you don't feel anything the first time, don't be discouraged. As I have said, it has been proven in energetic testing that even in the absence of a specific sensation, the energetic effect from the stones is still present. With a little patience and lots of listening with the body, the felt sense and the sensations will make themselves felt sooner or later.

For Children

Children can also take advantage of shungite's properties.

In general a child is well grounded and full of life. Unfortunately, however, the new technologies attract and overstimulate a child's upper chakras, especially with the overuse of computer games. Many children are overstimulated in the sixth chakra and this creates symptoms of hyperactivity. This syndrome can be understood energetically as an imbalance among the chakras and often a lack of grounding. The sixth chakra is greatly overdeveloped to the detriment of the first and seventh chakras (representing the mother and father respectively), which are too small.

Wearing a shungite pendant during the day (but not every day) and having harmonizers in the bedroom can, after a few weeks, help children get their bearings.

Shungite water, in small doses (half a glass in the morning), is also helpful for children. If they're sick you can increase the dose to one or two glasses a day.

For the Elderly

Shungite's ability to relieve pain through direct contact but also penetrating through any kind of material has led us to make belts or bands stuffed with shungite pebbles for use on the back, the waist, the knees, and so on.

The belts are helpful for people suffering from arthritis or pain due to aging. They can be worn in contact with the painful areas during the day and, if need be, also at night. Our personal experience has confirmed the effectiveness of these belts. Friends and clients have reported very positive results. The belts are placed against places that are painful or stiff in order to bring suppleness and mobility to the localized energy. They can also be worn against the kidneys in order to activate the whole energetic body, or in conjunction with walks or physical effort.

A carpet or cushion of shungite can be a good way to regain a bit of life force in elderly people. It can be used as a decorative piece on an armchair or sofa and will help the person rediscover a good alignment of the spinal column, reinforces strength and vigor, and relieves dorsal pain. Another way of using it is to take your shoes off and place your feet directly on it.

For those who have circulation problems in the lower limbs, varicose veins, or swollen feet, the shungite carpet will get the energy and the blood circulation moving again. It can be used for a few hours each day, but not in the two or three hours before bedtime since stimulation or activation before going to bed always should be avoided to obtain the benefit of a good night's sleep.

The shungite cushion can also be used to relieve, balance, and activate those confined to wheelchairs, whether their infirmity is temporary or ongoing. Moreover, this kind of cushion will protect the person from harmful radiation generated by motorized wheelchairs.

It is important to note that shungite should be used in

moderation in cases of hypertension. Shungite has a positive action on hypertension when scheduled competently with proper staging (as reported in accounts of the experiments conducted by Russian researchers). Overuse is never advisable.

Shungite in the Car and on Trips

When we spend time in vehicles, whether in a car or on public transit, we are cut off from the cosmic and telluric emanations of nature. Our bioenergetic measurements prove that just being seated in a closed automobile, without the motor running, shrinks our vital field by 15 percent compared to its normal extent. In addition, we are subjected to electromagnetic fields when the car's motor is running. With a GPS and a cell phone present, the interior of the vehicle becomes saturated with electromagnetic waves that have no way of escaping because the car acts like a Faraday cage. A Faraday cage is a metallic enclosure or cage that isolates a space against the influence of external electric fields while preventing any fields inside it from escaping.

Pulsed waves multiply inside a vehicle simply because, when the GPS or phone is operating, it is continually looking for networks as the vehicle moves from the signals of one relay tower to the next. The effect of a cell phone's emissions can be increased by up to a factor of ten inside a vehicle.

Everyone has felt the effect of a long car trip in which the fatigue is notably a result of the lack of contact with the ground and with the Earth. It is essential that you come back to your roots, to your presence, to your attention. Shungite is a big help in doing this. It reconnects us to the Earth, it recenters us, and protects us from the left torsion fields produced by motors and electromagnetic fields.

You can carry it on you in your pocket, as a pendant, or in a cloth belt. For people who use a vehicle daily or for long periods (taxi drivers or professional truck drivers) the best way to ward off harmful effects and fatigue is to put a shungite cushion on the driver's seat.

When traveling by plane, especially long-distance flights, the use of shungite (a necklace for example) helps us withstand the energetic disturbances caused by pressurization. When you arrive, keep the shungite on you for a little while because the grounding effect can help you get over the jet lag. When you get off the plane the first chakra is smaller. You need to reconnect with the ground on which you stand. Shungite reactivates this relationship. Make gifts of shungite to friends who are pilots or flight attendants—they will be very grateful to you!

The Shungite Room

A shungite room has recently been constructed in Paris. It is the first shungite room outside of Russia, and I hope that it will be the first of many others around the world. It's a room about 4 square meters (43 square feet). Its floor and walls are covered in shungite tiles and its ceiling contains a layer of powdered shungite. In order to provide a maximum level of relaxation, a comfortable armchair and shungite cushions round out the furnishings. The room is also designed so it can be completely black, without light, for certain energetic work.

As we saw in chapter 5, "Shungite Properties and Effects on Health," this kind of room has been shown to be a complementary therapeutic tool for harmonizing physiological, psychological, and energetic levels; for stimulating self-healing abilities; and for relaxing and spending a pleasant moment with oneself, while at the same time being protected from radiation and electromagnetic fields.

The room is used for 20-minute relaxation sessions in which the person lies down in the room and upon coming out receives a harmonization with the sounds of crystal singing bowls. Healers also come often to reenergize themselves and advise their clients to come to supplement other therapies.

This shungite room can also be used for carrying out numerous bioenergetic experiments. It's a unique opportunity that ushers in a new segment of bioenergetic research on shungite and will allow us to develop our experimentation projects further.

SHUNGITE AND DWELLING PLACES

Geobiology

Since the dawn of time, humans have aligned their needs with nature's energies. We built sacred spaces, as well as living quarters, while respecting and sometimes modifying the cosmic and telluric forces of places in order to adapt them vibrationally. Today this science, formerly used by shamans, Egyptians, Celts, Romans, and cathedral builders, is called *geobiology* in the West.

In our era, since most buildings are no longer based on ancestral knowledge, the bioenergetic equilibrium of our living spaces is no longer maintained. In any location where you spend several hours a day and especially in the places where you sleep and where you work, the expertise of a geobiology professional or a dowser can help you reestablish an optimal balance for your well-being and can reactivate your energy.

Shungite is beginning to be known and recognized in France among biogeologists who use it as an adjunct to their knowledge of the subtle energy domain. Shungite is not only useful for protecting against the electromagnetic fields that we have already enumerated but it is also a natural way of rebalancing cosmic and telluric energies.

Each biogeologist or dowser, of course, has their own personal techniques, but using shungite is beneficial for everyone since we're dealing with a totally natural substance with easily measurable bioenergetic effects. It can usefully round out the application of other means and other instruments in one's practice.

Be reminded that shungite never takes on a charge. Thus, using the appropriate form and caliber of shungite can cancel out or at least counterbalance the effect of a fault line or stray electric currents or other geopathic pollution.

Pyramids of shungite can be placed on a fault line, for example, at two ends of a room or house—at the places where the fault line enters and leaves, and at the center where the negative influence peaks—in order to eliminate the negative impact of the fault line on the energetic fields of the occupants. It is difficult to establish a scale for determining the dimensions of the pyramids to use since each fault line has a different effect depending on its intensity, its width, and its depth. All the variables of the fault and of the location to be protected must be taken into account. However, in my practice I have used two pyramids of shungite with 6 cm (2.4 inch) sides at each end of a living room that was 5 meters (16 feet) long and had an average fault line running through it. The fault line was causing a decrease of 30 percent of the vital field, a shift of the vertical plane 7 cm (2.8 inches) to the left, and a shift of the vertical plane 4 cm (1.6 inches) downward. These pyramids were enough to resolve the disturbances created by this fault line. A year later

I went back to check on my solution and I was pleased to see that the situation was stable and that the bioenergetic readings were still positive.

Obviously, with more powerful faults or with larger rooms it is necessary to use larger pyramids. It's important to remember that a shungite pyramid (or any other shape) placed on the high point of the disturbance will have its bioenergetic emanation reduced slightly.

It is clear that pyramids and other shungite objects can be used for any type of balancing and harmonization of negative waveforms and of lines and intersections of negative telluric networks. Nevertheless, I advise against the systematic use of pyramids, especially in bedrooms, because their energy and their waveforms are strong and do not go well with the "letting go" necessary for a good night's sleep. Some people suggest placing a pyramid under the bed thus eliminating the pollution once and for all. In doing so, the pollution will indeed be eliminated but you also risk not getting a proper rest, having a fitful sleep, or even insomnia.

For bedrooms, I advise using shungite spheres or eggs instead because, as I've already mentioned, their waveforms resonate more with our own bioenergetic fields.

In order to bring grounding to houses built on landfill, houses on pilings, and apartments on higher floors, the use of shungite cubes placed judiciously following the positive telluric networks will pull together the connection that the building was lacking. In this way the occupants of this type of locale are able to reestablish contact with the Earth. Shungite cubes can even be integrated into the construction of the home if your expertise can be applied before building begins.

BENEFICIAL INFLUENCE ZONES
FOR SPHERES AND PYRAMIDS PLACED
IN A NEUTRAL ZONE

Shungite Shape/Size	Influence Range
Pyramid: 5 cm (2 inches)	2.1–2.3 meters (6.9–7.5 feet)
Pyramid: 6 cm (2.4 inches)	2.5–2.7 meters (8.2–8.9 feet)
Pyramid: 7 cm (2.8 inches)	2.9–3.2 meters (9.5–10.5 feet)
Pyramid: 8 cm (3.1 inches)	3.5–3.9 meters (11.5–12.8 feet)
Pyramid: 9 cm (3.5 inches)	4.2–4.6 meters (13.8–15 feet)
Pyramid: 10 cm (3.9 inches)	5–5.4 meters (16.4–17.7 feet)
Sphere: 4 cm (1.6 inches)	2 meters (6.6 feet)
Sphere: 5 cm (2 inches)	2.7 meters (8.9 feet)
Sphere: 6 cm (2.4 inches)	3.65 meters (12 feet)
Sphere: 7 cm (2.8 inches)	5 meters (16.4 feet)
Sphere: 8 cm (3.1 inches)	6.6 meters (21.7 feet)
Sphere: 9 cm (3.5 inches)	8.9 meters (29.2 feet)
Sphere: 10 cm (3.9 inches)	12 meters (39.4 feet)

I need to stress that this table indicates the zone of influence of shungite objects placed in a neutral zone. As mentioned before, a shungite object that is placed in an area of disturbance will have its emanation reduced slightly in proportion to the intensity of the disturbance.

Harmonizing a Space

Even if you are not a geobiologist you can use shungite in your living quarters. Shungite objects such as pyramids, spheres, eggs, and cubes are designed for this purpose.

The fact that you are not aware of the disturbances present in your home is not a problem because shungite, unlike other stones and crystals, will not amplify disturbances but, on the contrary, balances them.

Based on my experience as a geobiologist, I have come to realize that certain stones have been used unwisely. I have seen large black tourmalines weighing 10–15 kg (22–33 lbs) in bedrooms. Of course, the occupants had trouble sleeping and even had frequent nightmares because the energy was too telluric.

I have also seen completely saturated rock crystal placed on negative telluric networks. Once a crystal is charged, or even saturated, the influence it sends out is the opposite of what is expected: it reemits the negative data through the force of its crystalline structure. A crystal that is saturated with a negative force sends out this information to a greater distance than if the crystal was not there.

I was also able to study the energetic effect of salt lamps and the effect of a crystal placed on a lamp or on a powerful electric source. The sole effect of these practices is to propagate the electromagnetic fields even farther. That doesn't happen with nonelectric salt lamps containing candles, which in contrast are positive. It's always possible to restore a positive effect to electric salt lights and to crystals placed right beside an electric source by protecting them with a shungite base.

There is no risk of making this kind of mistake with shungite because one of its characteristics is, and I can't repeat it often enough, to never become saturated or charged negatively.

The only risk there can be with shungite is to use too much of it by trying to overdo the protection or using it in an exaggerated way. Don't shut yourself up in a cage that is "anti-everything." Life is meant to be lived. Find the inner strength to face the situations that your existence brings you. Exaggerating the need for protection is not good.

Harmony is made up of subtle shades and the stones are there to accompany us in our experience of life, not to shut us away. For example, you can decide to fill your house with great quantities of stones and crystals which give off only very high spiritual vibrations. That way you will be living in a very high vibration environment, but when you have to go out the world is going to seem dull or, more likely, heavy. You can decide to completely neutralize all electromagnetic waves in your home, somewhat like making it into an electromagnetically insulated sealed chamber. But if you do that the world outside is going to feel extremely aggressive. That's not what lithotherapy is trying to accomplish.

If you want, you can create a restful place in your home, a personal relaxation space—your temple. A bit of shungite positioned in this space will neutralize the negative influences and other stones will contribute their characteristics depending on what you want to create: well-being, relaxation, gentleness, joy, or spiritual and energetic alignment. There are also harmonizers designed to produce various relaxing effects.

In bedrooms it is always better to use gentle forms such as spheres and eggs, as I have mentioned several times throughout this book. Other touches can be added with minerals such as selenite, amethyst, lepidolite, charoite, rose quartz, or white jade. These stones foster harmonization and overall balance so that elevated vibrations from the upper chakras can be received without stirring up the turning mind.

In living rooms, having a beautiful, large pyramid or a large sphere of shungite activates the space and permeates it with a revitalizing influence.

In offices, the priority is to balance the electromagnetic fields of all the electric and electronic equipment as we have outlined in the chapter devoted to this equipment. However, in order to stimulate quickness in the mind and to facilitate intellectual work, you can complement the shungite with rock crystal or fluorite.

If you already have big crystals, you can also place them on stands or plates made of shungite. That way you can avoid having to regularly purify or clear them since shungite has the ability to confer its capacity of not taking on a charge to stones placed on it.

SHUNGITE USE BY THERAPISTS

As therapists you are certainly aware of the importance of your energetic state when working with clients, regardless of the type of therapy you conduct.

Some sessions can be particularly difficult, tiring, challenging, exhausting, or even unbalancing. Being well grounded and at the same time open to subtle impressions is of utmost importance. It is sometimes necessary to recharge your energetic potential. Shungite is a quick and effective way of doing that.

The therapist's use of shungite harmonizers before the session, between sessions, or at the end of the day can provide reconnection with the therapist's own center while the energetic body is reinforced and reactivated. A quick rebalancing takes place in the proper alignment of polarities. All of these effects can help reinforce the healing energy that is afterward transmitted to the client.

Shungite harmonizers can also be offered to clients at the end of a session in order to help in the process of integration of information arrived at during therapy. This brief moment of meditation helps the transition from the therapeutic session back into the activities of everyday life.

A shungite pendant can also be worn by the therapist during the day. It will help you to stay energized, will quickly correct negative energetic influences, and will keep you connected to the Earth.

I have personally experienced an interesting effect with a shungite cushion during my bioenergetic working sessions. One day I placed one of these cushions on a chair in my office so someone could try it and then I forgot about it. During a workshop with several participants, the chair with the shungite cushion (which looked like all the other chairs) got placed at my desk without me knowing it. A couple of weeks later I was reflecting that the sessions of the recent period were particularly rich and effective, the quality of the information was subtle, and my work with clients had increased. A few days later, I realized that I had been sitting on the shungite cushion. Since then I can assure you the shungite cushion has remained on my chair.

In conclusion, I would also like to mention the fact that there are massage rods made of shungite, which are practical tools for those doing massage or for therapies based on the stimulation of energy points. The qualities of shungite already extensively described are totally applicable to this tool as well.

It is clear that shungite, because of its quality as the "stone of life," as well as many other stones and crystals that emanate beneficent energy, are always a welcome addition to a therapist's office simply by their very presence. If your office has equipment that is electric or uses pulsed waves (such as cordless phones), the negative energy of these radiations can be transformed with shungite.

8

SHUNGITE AND
OTHER STONES

No doubt you are already convinced about shungite's importance in lithotherapy, but that is not all: there is another quality of this amazing stone: shungite is a powerful catalyst.

Catalysis consists of using one substance, shungite in this case, with a reactive agent (any other stone or crystal used in lithotherapy) in order to speed up a reaction. Using a crystal combined with shungite activates and increases the effect of the crystal in its subtle interaction with the energetic body, deepening the impact of these effects. As we have already seen, this property has been applied to the principle of harmonizers, which work by moving energy based on a difference in potential. Shungite catalysis does not modify the catalyst and in addition, through its action on the first chakra, fosters the integration of the energetic process induced by the crystal.

In the course of my bioenergetic research I have experimented with numerous stones and over the years I became accustomed to meditating with stones and crystals in order to know them in their innermost depths. Since shungite has come into my life, it has changed my perception of the mineral world. It has contributed to the awakening of my ability to contact crystalline structures and to be able to take note of and recognize, through a simple contact, a vibratory signature belonging to a stone or a crystal.

In certain shamanic traditions and in certain traditional medicine systems, they speak of plants that teach or animal guides. I believe that such teachers exist in the mineral world. Through my own experience, I consider shungite to be a teaching stone and I invite you to experience it for yourself.

For those who are already expert in relating to stones, I am certain that you can experience stimulating adventures in shungite's company. Meditating with a piece of silver shungite associated with another stone can guide you to very profound discoveries and very rich teachings. You can use shungite as a therapeutic accompaniment, if you like, and you can recommend its catalyzing role with other stones and crystals according to the energetic needs of your client.

For those of you who are just beginning to discover the magnificent world of minerals and lithotherapy, shungite is a wonderful portal. The fact that shungite doesn't take on a charge facilitates the beginner's approach. We always recommend beginning with the base. Since shungite stimulates the first chakra and, in doing so, stabilizes our energetic body it safely opens the door to the exploration of the higher chakras.

Beginners in lithotherapy often wonder how they can know if crystals are negatively charged and how to release these charges.

This question is in fact not so simple and can even raise doubts about the relevance of one's own felt sense. I found a smart way around that problem by using a square shungite plate with sides of 10 cm (3.9 inches). I programmed in it an energetic accelerator specifically designed to remove the charge from all the other stones and realign them to their own natural vibration. The shungite always stays active and fosters the alignment of other crystals without becoming charged itself because that is one of its natural characteristics.

Other experiments with crystals have led me to put together new combinations of very effective harmonizers that extend their vibratory qualities to various energetic planes. The following list identifies some of these combinations, the chakras they influence, and the uses for which they can be employed.

- **Shungite and carnelian harmonizers (first and second chakras)**—for those who want to stimulate their creativity, regain a good relationship with their body and their sexuality, and develop their capacity to sense.
- **Shungite and tiger's eye harmonizers (first and third chakras)**—for those who are unsure of their abilities, lack courage in getting going, and can't find where they belong.
- **Shungite and rose quartz harmonizers (first and fourth chakras)**—for those who are easily destabilized by emotions; for those whose heart wants to regain its rightful place; and for those who want to regain a well-centered calm.
- **Shungite and blue calcite harmonizers (first and fifth chakras)**—for those who aren't sure they're on the right path; and for those who want to speak their own truth clearly.
- **Shungite and fluorite harmonizers (first and sixth chakras)**—for those who have lots of ideas but who have

trouble putting them in order; for students who have to digest a variety of intellectual information; and for generally promoting a good balance between the two hemispheres of the brain.

- **Shungite and rock crystal harmonizers (first and sixth chakras)**—for crystal experts who want to reach new subtle knowledge. By bringing together the carbon of shungite and the silica of rock crystal we have two teaching stones.

- **Shungite and selenite harmonizers (first and sixth chakras)**—for those who are often stressed and nervous; for returning to mental calm; for gently quieting a space (apartment, therapy office, business office).

- **Shungite and amethyst harmonizers (first and seventh chakras)**—this great pair works at aligning the energetic body, rooting in the peaceful energy from the high violet vibrations of the amethyst.

The catalyzing properties of shungite can also work in the preparation of shungite water with other stones and crystals.

9

SHUNGITE AND AGRICULTURE

Shungite can have numerous applications in agriculture, viticulture, and horticulture that extend equally well to garden plants and house plants, as well as fruit trees, vineyards, and even grain crops.

The frequent use of chemical fertilizers ends up making the fields toxic in the long run, weakening the natural nutritive value of the soil, and resulting in a significant reduction of organic material—the biomass. Fortunately, many farmers are turning toward other methods of farming that are more respectful of the environment and of themselves; either by finding alternative solutions or by moving to organic farming or biodynamic agriculture. Shungite can contribute certain solutions for a healthier agriculture. (See plate 12 of the color insert for a photo of shungite used in agriculture.)

First of all, shungite absorbs and neutralizes harmful chemicals, such as residues from pesticides, herbicides, fungicides, and other defoliants. We know that various chemical products being spread on fields do not decompose at the end of their period of usefulness. Therefore, a significant amount of these chemical compounds remains in the soil. Certain elements that are not leached away by precipitation or absorbed by deeper layers of earth remain and accumulate on the surface year after year. Shungite, because of the fullerenes that it contains (and the peculiarities of their molecular composition), attracts these toxic substances and neutralizes most of them.

We have seen that shungite stimulates what is living. Using shungite on the fields supports the rebuilding of the substrate of microorganisms that are naturally present in soil so that there is at least a partial return to a balanced, living structure in the fields and in the farming process. Experiments in Russia on large plots of farmland had satisfactory results with the introduction of 10 grams (0.4 ounces) per square meter (11 square feet) of land.

Having shungite present in water reservoirs used for agriculture (tanks, cisterns) or in the irrigation systems allows large-scale irrigation with shungite water.

FRENCH RESEARCH RESULTS

A study of the application of shungite on plants is now being carried out in France for over a year by Jean-Michel Pasternak and Claude Bernard. They sent me the following conclusions: "The tests conducted this year show a great tonicity in the plants, more vibrant colors, significant growth, and an accumulated resistance to blight and dryness."

They have established protocols in arboriculture relative to the quantities and timing of shungite watering or spreading it in pulverized form intended to enrich the substrates. They have also conducted experiments on the way foliage and roots absorb the shungite. Here is their advice:

Watering: Prepare three days in advance, add 5 liters (1.3 gallons) of water to a bucket with 1 to 1.5 kg. (2.2 to 3.3 pounds) of shungite in mineral form on the bottom. Use this water directly on your plants for watering. Or add 7 grams (0.25 ounces) of shungite powder for each liter (34 fluid ounces) of water and sprinkle it directly on plants.

For the substrates: You can mix in the shungite in order to improve the action of the mineral on the plants. Add 1 kg (2.2 pounds) of powdered shungite per cubic meter (35 cubic feet) of substrate to be used as is.

For restructuring the soil and promoting the elimination of toxic substances: Add 1 kg (2.2 pounds) of powdered or crushed shungite for each cubic meter (35 cubic feet) of substrate. Nine cubic meters (318 cubic feet) per hectare (2.5 acres) of this mixture is enough to restore balance to the soil. This spreading of shungite should be done once every two years.

For enriching a hectare (2.5 acres) of cultivated land: Add 1 kg (2.2 pounds) of powdered shungite per cubic meter (35 cubic feet) of substrate to be used as is. This spreading should be done once every three years.

Spreading on the soil: Add 30 to 40 grams (1.0 to 1.4 ounces) of semicrushed shungite per square meter (1.2 square yards) of soil. This spreading is done once every two to four years depending on the state of the soil.

USE ON FRUIT TREES AND SHRUBS

Remarkable results are obtained using shungite on fruit trees whether they're young plants or mature, fruit-bearing trees.

Several methods can be used:

- Add crushed shungite to the soil at the foot of the tree, or in the earth when the seedling is being planted.
- Spread powdered shungite at the foot of the tree.
- Water the orchards with shungite water.

Experiments carried out in both Russia and in France report a better root system in the plants, a reinforcement of natural defenses—and therefore a very good resistance against parasites— plus improved growth.

USE IN MARKET GARDENING

Since shungite promotes soil fertility, it is advised to spread crushed shungite in February, March, or April according to the planting season, and again after harvest. The amount of crushed shungite to apply is in the range 0.02 to 0.5 kg per square meter (0.04 to 1.1 pounds per 1.2 square yards) according to need, the characteristics of the particular soil, and the specific requirements of each type of planting.

You will notice right away a decrease in water consumption (shungite supports humidity retention), a reduction in the need to use chemicals (in the case of nonorganic farming), and enhanced productivity. Russian farmers have noticed an improved productivity in market gardening of between 20 percent and 40 percent!

In greenhouses, spreading a layer of shungite promotes photosynthesis and the black color raises, but also regulates, the temperature of the soil from the absorption of solar energy. We have seen that shungite exerts a thermic action on the cells so that they don't overheat. It works the same way with the plants; shungite receives and stores the sun's heat, passing it on to the plants and the soil in a continuous flow. Shungite also promotes humidity retention, thus reducing evaporation and lessening the need for irrigation.

Shungite powder can also be used as a component in the substrate used for hydroponic gardening.

USE WITH INDOOR PLANTS

The crushed stone is used both for water drainage and for the fertilization of indoor plants. You only need about 20 grams (0.7 ounce) of crushed shungite for 1 kg (2.2 pounds) of soil. Watering with shungite water is very good for potted plants; their luster and color change, which indicates that the plant is healthier in general and has increased vitality. You will also notice growth and significant development in the stems, leaves, and flowers.

You can conduct a very simple experiment by adding shungite to a vase of cut flowers: you will see that the flowers last longer and fade much less quickly.

CONCLUSION

Even though I am one of the pioneers in the use of shungite in France, the research presented here is far from being definitive. This book is simply a first stage in allowing a larger public to benefit from a wide-ranging spectrum of information about this stone that is beginning to charm more and more people.

In a few years perhaps researchers will have discovered other aspects of natural fullerenes and will be able to shed more light on how they came to be present in shungite. In 2011, having a shungite room makes a new research facility possible. A series of tests on the biochemistry of shungite water is also planned and tests on the application of shungite to agriculture will intensify.

As a final stage in our journey and by way of concluding, I propose to offer a "vibratory" point of view. Shungite resonates with the subtle frequency of the first chakra's red color, with the subtle frequency black in its link to the density of the Earth, and with the subtle frequency magenta of the magenta chakra—this chakra is found about 30 centimeters (1 foot) above the top of the head. These three frequencies engender a particular energetic movement that is very fine and at the same time very powerful.

The highest frequency present in shungite (the magenta frequency) is likely provided by the fullerene molecules. Contact with the magenta frequency allows us to be connected to the movement of life while contact with the other frequencies (red and black) is connected to the structure and basis of life. Because of these three frequencies, we can say that contact with shungite connects us to our *energy of life*.

TESTS

Shungite and Electromagnetic Waves

These tests were conducted with the collaboration of Christel Barbier, bioenergeticist and geobiologist.

In carrying out this study we have measured the energetic emanation of the body, the vital field and its sublayers, and the emanations of the chakras. The drawings that follow have been created using this measurement method. We took as a reference example a person (male) with a balanced energetic system (an average case as found in our bioenergetic practice). We positioned this person at a distance of 50 cm (1.6 feet) from a Wi-Fi hot spot, at 100 cm (3.3 feet) from a cordless phone base, in contact with a portable computer, and with a cell phone. Each of these measurements was noted and compared with the reference profile.

A number of parameters were measured:

• The dimensions of the vital field envelope
• The length of the chakras
• Positioning of the vital field axes
• Concentration of the vital field

The following should be kept in mind when evaluating the results:

- The smaller the vital field becomes, the more the body is being subjected to a disturbance. The larger it becomes, the more the body is functioning properly.
- The smaller the chakras become, the more the disturbance interferes with psychic and spiritual development.
- The more the vital field's vertical axis is shifted left in relation to the axis of the physical body, the worse the person feels and the more the disturbance has an effect on the body.
- The more the permeability of the vital field increases, the more the person is being subjected to a disturbance.

The choice of protection can be divided into two distinct systems: wearing a protection on the body or changing the signal emitted by the equipment with a localized protection. In the first case we are modifying the parameters of our own bioenergetic system by using a stone that increases its concentration through reinforcing the first chakra. This method allows our own bioenergetic system to continuously correct the harmful interference. In the second case, we are applying directly to the source of the disturbance information that corrects and transforms the electromagnetic waves into biocompatible emanations. So, in the case of pulsed electromagnetic waves (Wi-Fi, cordless phones, and cell phones) the corrected information will radiate with the same power as the original source of the disturbance but in a version that is positive and biocompatible.

SERIES OF WI-FI TESTS

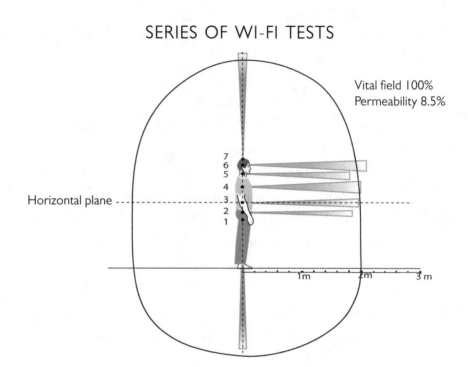

Vital field 100%
Permeability 8.5%

Horizontal plane

1m 2m 3 m

Reference profile of subject in a neutral zone.

The vital field envelope retracts by 25% and the chakras shrink by 30% to 40% (especially chakras one, four, and five). The only chakra that resists is the sixth—mental activity. The vertical axis is shifted 7 cm (2.8 inches) and the permeability is twice as great, which makes the person more sensitive to disturbances.

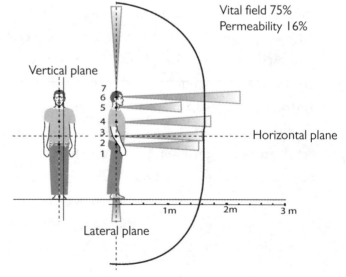

Vital field 75%
Permeability 16%

Vertical plane

Horizontal plane

Lateral plane

1m 2m 3 m

Profile of subject with a Wi-Fi hot spot 50 cm (1.6 feet) away.

The presence of the black tourmaline partially corrects the Wi-Fi hot spot signal. The person loses only 13% of the vital field and the vertical plane is only shifted 3 cm (1.2 inches). Notice the big increase in the first chakra which supports a better elimination of the disturbance and an increase in concentration of the field.

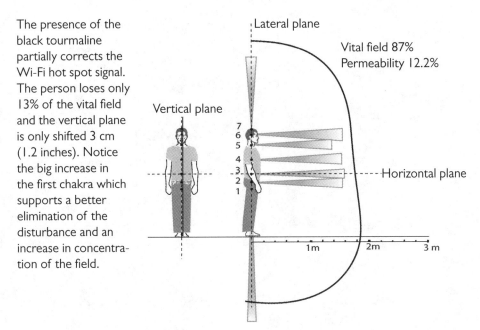

Profile of subject with a Wi-Fi hot spot 50 cm (1.6 feet) away, protected by a black tourmaline.

After seven weeks the tourmaline is saturated by the electromagnetic waves and, from that moment on, it begins to emit negative information. After three months, the disturbance is such that the effect on the person is more negative than without the protection.

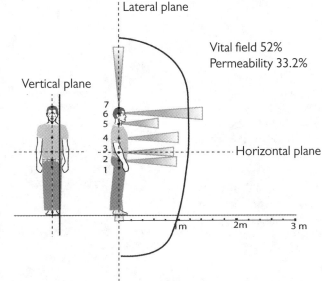

Profile of subject with a Wi-Fi hot spot 50 cm (1.6 feet) away, protected by a black tourmaline that has not been cleaned for three months.

Rock crystal protection means you lose only 10% of the vital field. The emanation of the crystal on the hot spot helps keep a balance between cosmic and telluric energy. The crystal takes on a charge after ten weeks and turns negative after four months.

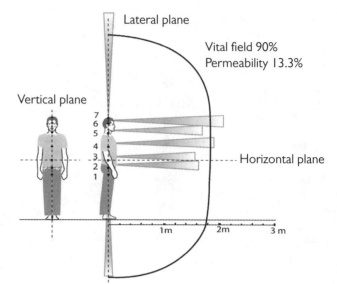

Profile of subject with a Wi-Fi hot spot 50 cm (1.6 feet) away, protected by a piece of rock crystal.

With the very significant contribution of energy from the crystalized hematite, the vital field increases by 10% over that of the reference profile. Most of the chakras increase. The permeability becomes almost normal thanks to a large first chakra. The stone begins to take on a charge at the end of ten months.

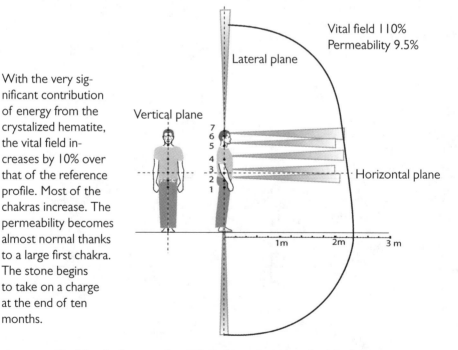

Profile of subject with a Wi-Fi hot spot 50 cm (1.6 feet) away, protected by a crystalized hematite.

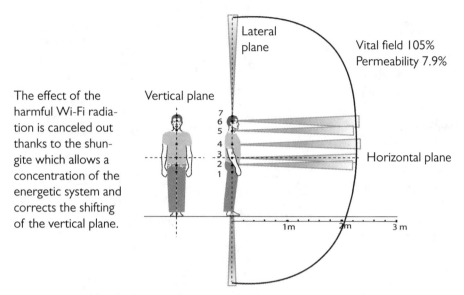

The effect of the harmful Wi-Fi radiation is canceled out thanks to the shungite which allows a concentration of the energetic system and corrects the shifting of the vertical plane.

Lateral plane

Vertical plane

Vital field 105%
Permeability 7.9%

Horizontal plane

1m   2m   3 m

*Profile of subject with a Wi-Fi hot spot 50 cm (1.6 feet) away,
protected by shungite.*

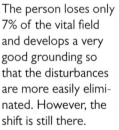
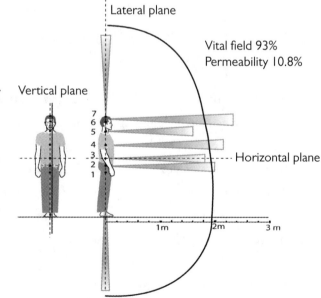

The person loses only 7% of the vital field and develops a very good grounding so that the disturbances are more easily eliminated. However, the shift is still there.

Lateral plane

Vertical plane

Vital field 93%
Permeability 10.8%

Horizontal plane

1m   2m   3 m

*Profile of subject with a Wi-Fi hot spot 50 cm (1.6 feet) away,
protected by a black tourmaline in the pocket.*

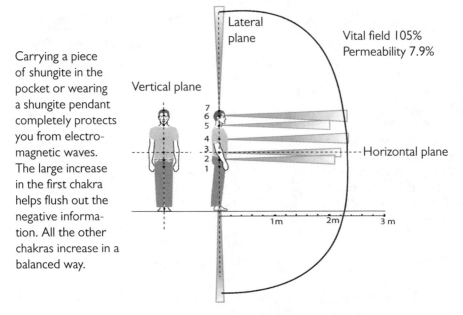

Carrying a piece of shungite in the pocket or wearing a shungite pendant completely protects you from electromagnetic waves. The large increase in the first chakra helps flush out the negative information. All the other chakras increase in a balanced way.

Profile of subject with a Wi-Fi hot spot 50 cm (1.6 feet) away,
protected by a piece of shungite in the pocket or a shungite pendant.

CONCLUSIONS
FROM THE WI-FI TESTS

In this first round of tests, we have studied a large number of different situations in order to show how the stones act and evaluate their effects from both a quantitative and qualitative point of view with respect to correction and protection.

Black tourmaline, often considered to be the best stone for protection against harmful radiation, didn't respond all that positively in our tests. It was almost surpassed by rock crystal's capacity to bring balance (comparing stones of equal weight). For personal protection, it's best to carry black tourmaline in your pocket (avoid pendants or necklaces of tourmaline, which have a crushing effect on the upper chakras). By looking at the diagrams, you can see that shungite and crystalized hematite are powerful protection stones since they completely correct the negative signal and they increase vital energy. Shungite, in addition, has the advantage of never taking on a charge. When you're on the move and find yourself in places that are polluted with electromagnetic waves from sources you cannot correct, you can either carry shungite in your pocket or you can wear a shungite pendant. Note that by placing shungite on a Wi-Fi source, your vital field will increase 5 percent because the positive information is carried by pulsed waves that have been made biocompatible.

SERIES OF CORDLESS PHONE TESTS

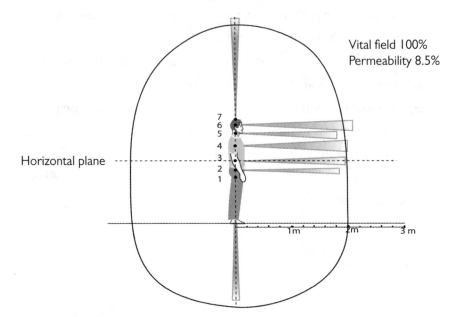

Vital field 100%
Permeability 8.5%

Horizontal plane

Reference profile in a neutral zone.

The vital field enve-
lope retracts by 25%,
the chakras shrink by
30% to 40% (especial-
ly chakras one, four,
and five). The only
chakra that resists
is the sixth—mental
activity. The vertical
axis is shifted 7 cm
(2.8 inches) and the
permeability is twice
as great which makes
the person more sen-
sitive to disturbances.

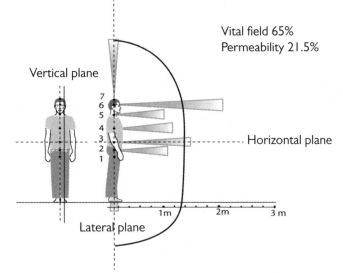

Vertical plane

Vital field 65%
Permeability 21.5%

Horizontal plane

Lateral plane

Profile of subject with a cordless phone base (DECT) 1 meter
(1.09 yards) away.

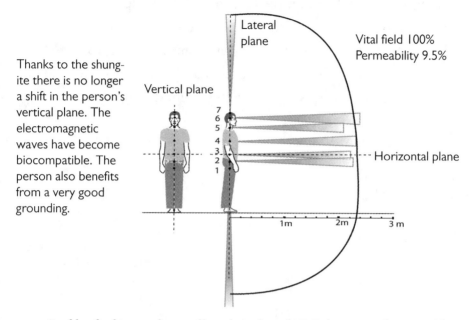

Thanks to the shungite there is no longer a shift in the person's vertical plane. The electromagnetic waves have become biocompatible. The person also benefits from a very good grounding.

Profile of subject with a cordless phone base (DECT) 1 meter (1.09 yards) away, protected by a piece of shungite.

CONCLUSIONS FROM THE CORDLESS PHONE TESTS (DECT)

In this series of tests, we are presenting only the tests with shungite. Tests carried out with other stones had results very close to those carried out with Wi-Fi.

Cordless phones are among the most powerful disturbances in our immediate environment (home and office), and at the same time they are the least recognized. As you can see in the diagram, the vital field decreases by 35 percent and the permeability skyrockets. The effects are just as bad when you are on the phone; subjecting you to significant disturbance even when you are far from the base. Black tourmaline hardly corrects the effects at all. Shungite placed on the base, or a shungite sphere or pyramid nearby, gives very good results by completely correcting all harmful effects. Also, once the signal from the base is corrected by shungite, you will enjoy the benefits of this new influence and your energy will increase by up to 20 percent during the call.

SERIES OF COMPUTER TESTS

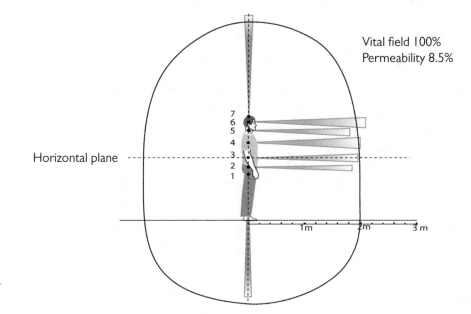

Horizontal plane

Vital field 100%
Permeability 8.5%

Reference profile in a neutral zone.

When we work on a portable computer, we lose 30% of the vital field and the vertical plane is shifted 12 cm (4.7 inches). Mental activity (sixth chakra) is stimulated excessively to the detriment of the overall energetic system. Because of the loss of vitality that results, we can become nervous and irritable.

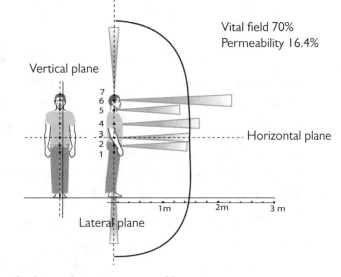

Vertical plane

Vital field 70%
Permeability 16.4%

Horizontal plane

Lateral plane

Profile of subject when using a portable computer.

You can use a shungite stone or a shungite plate designed for this use in order to rebalance the harmful effects of working on a portable computer. The concentration of your vital field will increase and your tiredness will decrease.

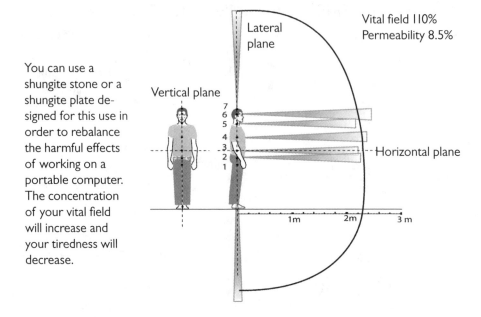

Profile of subject when using a portable computer protected with shungite.

CONCLUSIONS FROM THE COMPUTER TESTS

For this series of tests, we used a 15-inch portable computer of average configuration. The person tested had their hands on the keyboard, the usual position in which users spend hours every day. The loss of energy is 30 percent and the seventh and fifth chakras (awareness and communication, expression) were strongly disturbed, giving rise to feelings of depletion and exhaustion in users who spend long periods at the computer. The following are the most effective solutions that we recommend from among the stones tested.

Shungite, which fully corrects the transmission, can be easily transported and placed on all models of computers. It is equally effective on desktop computers. By placing it on the tower, it completely alters the transmission including keyboard and mouse. Shungite increases the vital field by 10 percent (after being applied). Shungite can be used in its form as an untreated stone (type I, silver quality) or a polished, tumbled stone or as a plate to be placed on the computer. Its power to concentrate and activate makes this stone a real panacea to be used with electromagnetic equipment, especially because it does not take on a charge.

Black tourmaline and rock crystal, in contrast, as in the tests on Wi-Fi, do not completely transform the disturbances arising from the computer and they become charged after being used for a certain period of time. If the user is unable, using bioenergetic measurement or radiesthesia, to determine their state of being charged, it is better not to use these stones. Otherwise, you run the risk of being subjected to a negative radiation that is multiplied by the stone's emanation, causing the opposite effect of what you are trying to accomplish.

By carrying a piece of shungite in your pocket (or wearing a pendant), the vital field only loses 5 percent and the permeability is at 9.7 percent, which is a good solution in a work situation or when it's not possible to directly alter computer radiation.

SERIES OF CELL PHONE TESTS

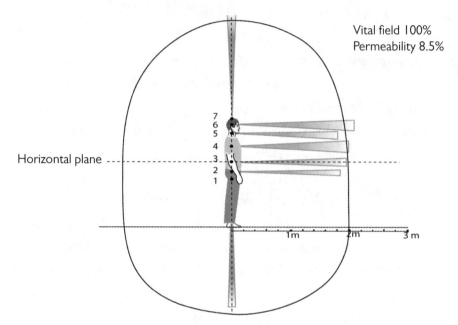

Vital field 100%
Permeability 8.5%

Horizontal plane

7
6
5
4
3
2
1

1m   2m   3 m

Reference profile in a neutral zone.

We see a vertical shift of 22 cm (8.7 inches) at the level of the head and the vital field decreases by 40%. The sixth chakra stays very active with an illusory sense of being more able to control things; the mind is overactive.

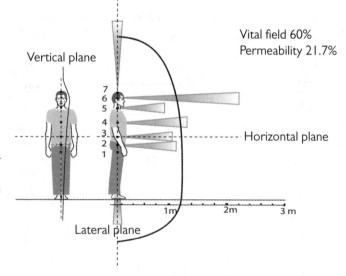

Vital field 60%
Permeability 21.7%

Vertical plane

Horizontal plane

7
6
5
4
3
2
1

1m   2m   3 m

Lateral plane

Profile of subject while on a cell phone call.

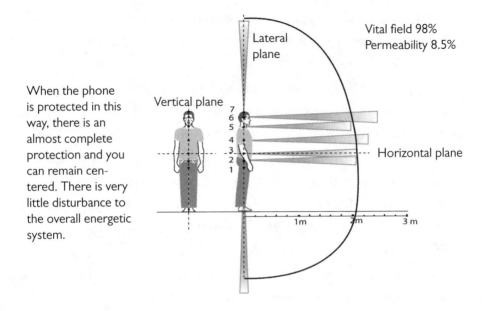

When the phone is protected in this way, there is an almost complete protection and you can remain centered. There is very little disturbance to the overall energetic system.

Profile of subject while on a cell phone call with the phone protected with a shungite patch.

CONCLUSIONS FROM THE CELL PHONE TESTS

Cell phones are now part of daily life and are used without a second thought by children and adolescents not only for communication but for music and photography. However, these ordinary everyday things are a permanent source of pulsed electromagnetic waves and affect the integrity of our energetic bodies.

Several medical investigations are underway to determine if cell phones are really harmful to the physical body. This testing encounters difficulties because the protocols that must be put in place are laborious and long-term.

We have used protocols with different scales relating to energetic testing and we have determined that the energetic system is highly disturbed by exposure to this type of wave; even more so because of how close the body is to the source of radiation.

As the diagrams from the tests make clear, when you are on a cell phone call, you undergo a loss of 40 percent of your energy, the energetic body becomes very permeable, and the only chakra that is not decreased is the sixth chakra (the mind chakra). This means that all the energy goes into the head, while the fifth chakra (throat) which is the subtle area of communication is severely reduced. The shift in the vertical plane is also significant at the level of the head and shows how the action is localized. All of these disturbances in the energetic field remain active for a certain time after the end of the call. The time required for a return to a normal state depends on the length of the call.

We tested the shungite patch that sticks onto the phone as a remedy for these negative effects. It returns the vital field to its correct concentration and protects the energetic body during a cell phone call.

BIOELECTROGRAPHIC TESTS USING GVD CAPTURE

By Stéphane Cardinaux

Bioelectrography is a measurement technique based on the Kirlian effect and perfected by Professor Korotkov. The principle of the GDV (Gas Discharge Visualization) measurement apparatus is the capture of an electrophotonic image; that is, through the amplification of photons emitted by the cells when they are subjected to a high voltage but very weak intensity electric field. Using this apparatus, an image is generated by computer, based on each of your ten fingers, showing the overall energy level of your systems and organs.

Various software applications then allow you to see your vital field (front or profile views), thus providing a comprehensive picture of the balance of the sympathetic and parasympathetic parts of the autonomic nervous system.

A diagram allows you to evaluate the level of stress in organs and systems, and to compare their level to that of a healthy person. You are given an overall picture of the areas of energetic deficiency, excess, or stagnation.

A virtual representation of the chakras allows a link to be established between blocked emotions and the system of thought. Generally, this representation is an excellent summary of present-day problems and problems from the past. It is ideal for comparing people, as well as measuring the effect of a therapy, a product, or a source of disturbance.

TESTS WITH SHUNGITE

The measurements carried out using the GDV apparatus are not intended to prove shungite's effects but to show what happens in the body when shungite is carried on one's person and how the energetic system reacts when it is subjected to a source of disturbance or to a product.

The first test concerns the effect of silver shungite.

Silver Shungite (Type I)
The results of this test are displayed in the shungite type I chart in the color insert (plate 13).

The chakra diagram shows that a person holding this type of shungite sees an increase in the reserve of vital energy at an emotional level, thereby providing a better buffer when confronted by external emotional aggression. The most striking effect is a better internal alignment, and therefore a greater ability to resist unbalancing forces. At the physical level, the alignment is also noticeable, but it's the net increase in the energetic and physical reserve which accounts for the major effect (see diagram with the measurements of energetic readings). Also notice how type I shungite aligns the first chakra. This is a clear sign of good grounding, a good contact with telluric energy.

The diagram of the organs summarizes the energetic level of more than fifty organs, systems, and glands. With type I shungite you see a balancing among the various organs. The smoothness of the curve (fewer hollows and bumps) is the sign of smoothness in the subtle energetic body.

Black Shungite (Type II)

The results of this test are displayed in the shungite type II chart in the color insert (plate 14).

The general idea of this test is to demonstrate shungite's influence as an agent that protects against harmful electromagnetic effects. To do this we used a type II shungite pyramid with a 7 cm (2.8 inches) base and a cordless phone (DECT) base to simulate the harmful disturbance.

Four measurements of the subject were taken: the first without doing anything; the second after turning on the cordless phone 20 cm (7.9 inches) away from the person being measured; the third with the pyramid placed beside the phone; and, finally, the fourth after turning off the phone and leaving the pyramid in place.

The effect of the electromagnetic field (7 V/m) is striking: it shifts all the chakras to the left (left torsion field effect), especially the lower three chakras, which has the effect of cutting the person off from their source of telluric energy. The third chakra, called the *energetic chakra,* is even the one that is shifted the most. We need to make clear that the person was measured standing while the phone was on a table and therefore closer to the lower chakras. It's likely that for a person sitting down, the fourth chakra would be somewhat more affected.

In positioning the pyramid, a few seconds was all it took to counter for the most part the effects of the harmful electromagnetic source. The first chakra regained its place in the energetic alignment. A few minor shifts remained but the overall energetic level of the chakras increased very clearly, a sign of a good energetic circulation between the lower and upper parts of the body. The energetic levels are compared in the bar chart of the measurements of the energetic levels in each phase of the test.

Once the power to the cordless phone base was turned off, only the effect of the shungite remains. Notice how the alignment comes back to the starting point (preliminary measurements), with a very slight increase in the energetic readings. You will notice that the shungite has more of an effect when the phone base is turned on. That may seem contradictory but it is easily explained by the torsion fields. The shungite actually emits a strong right torsion field that converts the phone's left torsion field into a right torsion field. The subtle component (etheric) of the electromagnetic energy gets combined with the etheric energy of the stone, thereby amplifying the overall effect.

I would like to make clear that, for this test, the person measured was sensitive and had good energy but was not particularly electrosensitive. The results of the measurements taken by the GDV apparatus were completely consistent with the felt sense of the person during the experiment: a sense of disturbed left/right balance as soon as the phone was turned on, a centering effect when the pyramid was put in place, and a sensation of energetic circulation all along the spinal column.

Although the GDV measurement protocol was rigorous, these tests need to be conducted with a good dozen individuals and be blinded in order to have scientific validation. In my opinion, these few measurements are very promising and I have no doubt about the conclusions that I arrived at because they clearly tally, in the electronic measurements, with the felt sense of hundreds of people.

The tests described in this appendix were conducted by Stéphane Cardinaux in December 2010. As mentioned in the introduction to this book, Cardinaux is an EPFL architect. He is also a practitioner and trainer of geobiology and bioenergy and a specialist in GDV electrophotonic assessment. He runs training courses at his center, the Génie du Lieu in Switzerland, which he founded in 2000. Cardinaux has written a number of books, primarily in French, on the subject of sacred geometry, bioenergy, and geobiography.

APPENDIX III

SHUNGITE AND ELECTROSENSITIVITY

The Importance of the First Chakra

For some years now, the word *electrosensitivity* has appeared among the pantheon of new pathologies linked to our technological era. Some people identify themselves as electrosensitive, sometimes almost priding themselves on it, as if they want to escape from a situation that they cannot manage by claiming to be victims of harmful influences from certain aspects of technology. In a way, being electrosensitive reflects an objective reality, but it also represents being willingly confined to a medically recognized kind of category that leads to a certain isolation when you consider the implementation of solutions that are sometimes onerous and rather dramatic.

In speaking this way, I am not at all trying to negate the discomfort and suffering of those who are electrosensitive. I am only reading this phenomenon differently and attempting to bring to it my contribution toward a solution.

I have been practicing bioenergetics for some years now and, as I mentioned in chapter 6 of this book, I have conducted many personal assessments that involved comparing them statistically with my colleagues' assessments. What I discovered from this is that, without exception, all the patients who defined themselves as electrosensitive, or who complained of similar symptoms, had an energetic blockage at the level of the first chakra.

Electrosensitive people very often had already tried many solutions before contacting us. Some of these solutions could be costly—such as completely confining oneself away from the world in a room sheathed in aluminum, or never going out unless one wore protective mesh clothing. Other solutions included installing rather significant quantities of black tourmaline, labradorite, or both.

Let's be clear—shungite is not a new miracle cure that can take the place of or be added to other solutions even though the electromagnetic protection properties and functions of this mineral are really impressive.

Shungite is certainly an essential tool of electromagnetic protection and a contributor to the process of healing electrosensitivity. However, from my point of view, it is absolutely essential to go after the underlying causes of electrosensitivity and root them out. Healing must be supported by a personal process to which therapists are simply an aid, a support, and a kindly guidance in the direction of healing. Each electrosensitive individual needs to conduct a personal work of accepting the energy of the Earth, this energy of life that is free and permanently available. Such a person needs to once again find their own "grounding wire." What's needed then is to discover, analyze, and remove obstacles to the connections among thinking, emotions, and Earth energy or materiality.

The first chakra is the domain of the Earth, of concentration or density, of matter, of the archetypal mother, of your own mother, of blood, of lineage, and of your genealogical tree. It is also the domain of all materialization and security: your home, your money, and your own physical and material security. All the problems that you encounter related to these themes undermine the expression of the first chakra.

One of the consequences of this kind of difficulty is an escape into the higher, up toward the seventh chakra—a desire to flee from the material world and to go more and more toward the "light," toward the subtle and spiritual higher vibrations (and only those), and to be related to the angels and the beings of the subtler planes. In doing this, we forget, we neglect, and we completely abandon our incarnation, our physical body.

After a certain amount of time being engaged in this "flight to the higher," people become more and more permeable to all kinds of influences and they lack good grounding. Permeability to various influences creates a state of fear, which in turn shrinks the energetic field.

The creative power of the mind is great. It is the mind that creates our energetic blockages, but it is also the mind that can clarify them. A reintegration of our Earth energy is therefore essential for us to regain energetic balance.

Let's get back to electromagnetic pollution and to the tests that we conducted on this topic. We subjected a neutral (and willing) subject to these tests, someone who was unaware of the outcome of the Wi-Fi field emission test. As in the previous tests, we noticed a reduction of the vital field by 25 percent and a loss of concentration or density. Using a computer, we then showed the same person a chart of all the electromagnetic networks that were passing through this same location, pointing out to him how the combined effect of all this radiation was terribly harmful. In repeating the bioenergetic measurements on that individual, we found a reduction of 40 percent to 50 percent of the vital field. These tests (which we repeated several times with the same results) show how our mental processes play a determining role in the way we relate to our environment.

Harmony is found in the integration of the two polarities; yin and yang, ba and ka, light and darkness, the higher and the lower, the material and the subtle. A balanced alignment is consciousness.

I advise electrosensitive people therefore to regain their grounding. Methods you can use for this are to set aside for a time activities that stimulate strongly the upper chakras (sixth and seventh), and to accept that you have to find ways to work with the type of difficulty that the first chakra presents. We recommend that you drink shungite water and use shungite harmonizers to regain balance. Wearing a shungite pendant or necklace is also an option, but you have to know how to use it in moderation. In such cases shungite must be used as a support for regaining your bioenergetic balance and your innate protection and not as a supplementary protection weapon against attack from outside yourself. Finally, there are very simple exercises you can do, such as walking down the street or through the countryside and feeling the soles of your feet touch the ground at every step.

RESOURCES

For more information about shungite or to order shungite products, visit the author's website **www.shungite-protection-and-healing.com**.

Those readers who find themselves in Paris are welcome to visit the author's shop and experience the shungite room described in this book.

La Roche Mère
7 rue Gambey
75011 Paris

The author can be reached by e-mail at **contact@shungite-protection-and-healing.com**.

Shungite can also be ordered from the following sources:

AhhhMuse!
2340 Hwy 180 E. #171
Silver City, NM 88061
575-534-0410
mqt@AhhhMuse.com • Bridgette@AhhMuse.com
www.AhhhMuse.com

Heaven and Earth LLC

P.O. Box 249

East Montpelier, VT 05651

heavenandearth@earthlink.net

www.heavenandearthjewelry.com

Uriël Creations LLC

Karen Kaufman

P.O. Box 3085

Monument, CO 80132

602-292-6818

karen@urielcreations.com

www.urielcreations.com

SELECTED
BIBLIOGRAPHY

Alekseev, N. I., D. V. Afanas'ev, B. O. Bodyagin, A. K. Sirotkin, N. A. Charykov, and O. V. Arapov. "A Possible Mechanism of Formation of Fullerene Nanoparticles in Shungites." *Russian Journal of Applied Chemistry* 80, no. 1 (2006): 139–46.

Becker, Luann, Jeffrey L. Bada, Robert J. Poreda, and T. E. Bunch, "Extraterrestrial Helium (He@C60) Trapped in Fullerenes in the Sudbury Impact Structure" (abstract of meeting, Large Meteorite Impacts and Planetary Evolution, 1997). Lunar and Planetary Institute website, accessed August 20, 2013, www.lpi.usra.edu/meetings/impacts97/pdf/6079.pdf.

Buseck, Peter R., Semeon J. Tsipursky, and Robert Hettich. "Fullerenes from the Geological Environment." *Science* 257, no. 5067 (July 1992): 215–17.

Cami, Jan, Jeronimo Bernard-Salas, Els Peeters, and Sarah Elizabeth Malek. "Detection of C60 and C70 in a Young Planetary Nebula." *Science* 329, no. 5996 (September 2010): 1180–82.

Koshland, Daniel E., Jr. "Molecule of the Year." *Science* 254, no. 5039 (December 1991): 1705.

Kurotchencko, S. P., T. I. Subbotina, I. I. Tuktamyshev, I. Sh. Tuktamyshev, A. A. Khardartsev, and A. A. Yashin. "Shielding Effect of Mineral Schungite during Electromagnetic Irradiation of Rats." *Bulletin of Experimental Biology and Medicine* 136, no. 5 (November 2003): 458–59.

Parthasarathy, G., R. Srinivasan, M. Vairamani, K. Ravikumar, and A. C. Kunwar. "Occurrence of Fullerenes in Low Grade Metamorphosed Proterozoic Shungite in Karelia, Russia." *Geochimica et Cosmochimica Acta* 62, no. 21–22 (November 1998): 3541–44.

INDEX

Page numbers in *italics* refer to illustrations.

BOOKS OF RELATED INTEREST

Himalayan Salt Crystal Lamps
For Healing, Harmony, and Purification
by Clémence Lefèvre

Stone Medicine
A Chinese Medical Guide to Healing with Gems and Minerals
by Leslie J. Franks

The Clay Cure
Natural Healing from the Earth
by Ran Knishinsky

The Oil Pulling Miracle
Detoxify Simply and Effectively
Birgit Frohn

Colloidal Silver
The Natural Antibiotic
by Werner Kühni and Walter von Holst

Crystal Healing for the Heart
Gemstone Therapy for Physical, Emotional, and Spiritual Well-Being
by Nicholas Pearson

Crystals for Karmic Healing
Transform Your Future by Releasing Your Past
by Nicholas Pearson

The Healing Intelligence of Essential Oils
The Science of Advanced Aromatherapy
by Kurt Schnaubelt, Ph.D.

Inner Traditions • Bear & Company
P.O. Box 388
Rochester, VT 05767
1-800-246-8648
www.InnerTraditions.com

Or contact your local bookseller